Praise for

RADIANT REST

"Within this book lies the medicine the world most needs. In our stillness our salvation lies, and these words will get you there."

—KATE NORTHRUP
best-selling author of *Do Less*

"*Radiant Rest* is a heartfelt and transformative gift to a weary, traumatized world, urging us to take rest as a path of liberation. Tracee Stanley eloquently channels the blessings of this profound and necessary lineage into an accessible path of practice that embraces our most inclusive selves."

—LAMA ROD OWENS
author of *Love and Rage*, co-author of *Radical Dharma*

"A wise and beautiful call to honor rest as both our birthright and our portal to embodied intelligence. Tracee Stanley's *Radiant Rest* shares the transformative power of yoga nidra with beginners and advanced practitioners alike; this work is vital for our world today."

—ELENA BROWER
best-selling author of *Practice You*

"Tracee Stanley is the medicine woman who shows up when you're done with fast food personal growth and you're ready for spiritual nectar. Sourced from the ancients and Tracee's devotion, *Radiant Rest* is gorgeously counterculture—which is why it's so healing."

—DANIELLE LAPORTE

author of *The Desire Map* and *Heart Centered*

"Tracee's wisdom comes with an unparalleled level of depth and grace. Her grounded style of teaching allows your heart to open and soften so you can receive the transmission of deep healing, surrender, and inner peace. While these ancient teachings have stood the test of time, Tracee delivers them in a fresh way that feels somehow new, yet directly connected to the source from which they came. Prepare yourself to receive golden wisdom from a teacher who is deeply steeped in both practice and truth."

—SHANNON ALGEO

author of *Trust Your Truth,* host of *SoulFeed* podcast

"Tracee Stanley is a true embodiment of the promises held in the title of this book—*Radiant Rest.* Tracee possesses a sparkly calm that emanates from her capacity to anchor into the body and the kindness of the heart. Use her words and the practices of yoga nidra to deepen your own relationship to rest, pleasure, and the type of beauty that can only arise out of a true connection to the present-moment self. I am a huge fan."

—KATIE SILCOX

author of *New York Times*–best seller *Healthy Happy Sexy*,
founder of The Shakti School

RADIANT
· REST ·

YOGA NIDRA
for Deep Relaxation
& Awakened Clarity

TRACEE STANLEY

Illustrations by Maggie Eileen

SHAMBHALA

Shambhala Publications, Inc.
2129 13th Street
Boulder, Colorado 80302
www.shambhala.com

Library of Congress Cataloging-in-Publication Data
Names: Stanley, Tracee, author.
Title: Radiant Rest: Yoga Nidra for deep relaxation and awakened clarity / Tracee Stanley.
Description: First edition. | Boulder, Colorado: Shambhala, 2021. |
Includes bibliographical references.
Identifiers: LCCN 2020033041 | ISBN 9781611808551 (trade paperback)
Subjects: LCSH: Rest. | Relaxation.
Classification: LCC RA785 .S743 2021 | DDC 612.7/6—dc23
LC record available at https://lccn.loc.gov/2020033041

Now is the time
for you to learn how to sleep
& awaken to your power.

Contents

Conclusion: The True Secret to Freedom   167

Introduction

Yoga Nidra: Beyond Technique

Yoga nidra has been called many things. In Sanskrit, the word *nidra* translates as "sleep," and *yoga nidra* has become widely known as the "yoga of sleep." It is also described as conscious sleep, the sleep of the yogis, transcendent, cosmic, and Divine—all of which are true. Yet no matter how we try to capture the essence of yoga nidra, no words can truly transmit the magic and mystery of the practice. If you have ever floated in a sea of stars or felt that you have peered through a wormhole into another dimension during yoga nidra, you know what I mean.

The yoga pose *Savasana* (Corpse Pose) is done in a supine resting position, and yoga nidra is traditionally practiced in this pose. People in Savasana may look like they're sleeping, but if they have set the intention to practice yoga nidra, they have merely begun to prepare—there is much more going on.

The association with sleep has both positive and negative connotations. On the positive side, it makes the practice very attractive. Who doesn't want to lie down and sleep? Studies show that most of us sleep an average of one to two hours less per night than people did sixty years ago. The poor, single mothers and people in marginalized communities are at even greater risk of suffering from sleep deprivation. Not getting enough sleep causes more harm than just feeling tired; studies show that it can weaken overall immune function and general health. The association of yoga nidra with regular sleep is certainly one of the reasons the practice continues to gain popularity in our sleep-deprived, biohacking society.

If we reduce the practice of yoga nidra to something as simple as a kind of nap, we may never discover all the clarity and power that a devoted practice can awaken. Science continues to learn more about sleep—for example, how delta waves produced during sleep help to form long-term memories[1]—but so much is still shrouded in mystery. Just what did the *rishis* and *rishikas*, the original seers, know about the power of yoga nidra?

A growing number of important and powerful voices are urging people to rest, to do less, to move away from the toxic culture of grinding it out and crushing it. Rest is vital to thriving. We have gotten the message that we need to actively make time for rest, to take up space, and to clear and protect space for those who have been denied the ability to rest safely. When we practice yoga nidra, we not only experience the power of deep rest and relaxation, but we get to wake up to our essential nature, one that is filled with radiance and bliss. This awakening has lasting and transformative effects on every aspect of our lives. Deep rest is just one of the many gifts we receive from the practice of yoga nidra.

The word *nidra* has another meaning besides "sleep": *ni* means "void," and *dru* means "to draw forth or reveal."[2] Yet a void is unknowable; it has been described as both empty and full. Philosophers and poets have dedicated pages upon pages to this concept, one we can't quite grasp. Our journey toward the void requires us to surrender to the unknown. The Indian English poet, philosopher, and yogi Sri Aurobindo described the void in *The Life Divine*:

> A silence, an entry into a wide or even immense or infinite emptiness is part of the inner spiritual experience ... this silence is the silence of the spirit which is the condition of a greater knowledge, power and bliss, and this emptiness is the emptying of the cup of our natural being, a liberation of it from its turbid contents so that it may be filled with the wine of God; it is the passage not into non-existence but to a greater existence.[3]

The journey of yoga nidra is elusive; it can't be owned, commodified, or branded. It can only be experienced. Your practice is the teacher, a portal that will lead you deeper into who you are, your power and radiance. Just when you think you understand, something new will be revealed to you. This is the nature of consciousness, ever expanding.

Yoga nidra can be understood as a technique, a state of consciousness, and a Goddess. It is expansive, supportive, and nurturing, a powerful practice for anyone. Yet it transcends our ability to truly describe it, try as we might. If there is one thing I know it's that this is the practice we all deserve. And it's my passion for sharing a practice that holds so much promise to enrich your life, health, and spiritual transformation that propels me to humbly offer my understanding and personal experience of yoga nidra.

WAKING UP

Let's try to reframe our idea of yoga nidra, moving away from it as simply something to do or teach, just a technique. First let's consider the idea that yoga nidra is a state of consciousness that is said to be "peace beyond words." Even though I call myself a yoga nidra teacher, I am actually sharing the methods that can lead to the state of consciousness that is yoga nidra. Arriving at that state requires preparation, clarity, and grace.

The state of yoga nidra is not something you can force or demand. The beauty is that, during preparation (the techniques), you get to rest deeply and learn about true surrender by expanding your capacity to be held and supported. You may glimpse where and why you are stuck in repeating patterns. You become more peaceful and intuitive; you can amplify your clarity, creativity, self-knowledge, and feel empowered to claim your birthright to experience deep rest. You may allow yourself to fall asleep to all that is not real and lasting, such as the desire for fame and material wealth. You may wake up to the eternal and radiant part of yourself that is always watching, the part of you that knows and never sleeps. By practicing the "sleep of the yoginis," you can radically awaken to the magic and knowledge that the universe holds while most of the world is sleeping. This type of wakefulness is more important than ever if we truly want to be part of a change that creates a more beautiful and just world for everyone.

The Bhagavad Gita describes it in chapter 2, verse 69:

YĀ NIŚHĀ SARVA-BHŪTĀNĀṀ TASYĀṀ JĀGARTI SANYAMĪ
YASYĀṀ JĀGRATI BHŪTĀNI SĀ NIŚHĀ PAŚHYATO MUNEḤ
What all beings consider as day is the night of ignorance for the wise,
   and what all creatures see as night is the day for the introspective
   sage.

THE PROMISE OF YOGA NIDRA

I often begin classes in my retreats and workshops with an opening circle where I ask participants to share a few words about why they decided to attend. When I was doing research for this book, I shared the practices of deep relaxation and yoga nidra with more than six hundred people and held some version of an opening circle with them too. While many people shared that they desperately needed rest, an overwhelming number said they were also seeking clarity, a connection to their inner knowing, or purpose in life. Yoga nidra can help with all these things, which are in fact the milestones on the path toward spiritual freedom.

It is easy to forget that yoga is a spiritual practice when we are constantly bombarded on our social media feed with images of models doing yoga and selling the latest gadget. Consider this a reminder: yoga is a practice that can lead us to spiritual freedom, transcendence, and enlightenment, and the practice of yoga nidra is a full system of yoga. It is both the means to freedom and freedom itself. Keeping that in our hearts as we practice changes the trajectory of our practice and affects our lives in meaningful ways. Even though we may be "doing" a technique, it is no longer rote or systematic. We are not checked out or begging for a dark, heavy sleep to come. Our intention for practice is elevated to the desire for radiant rest and awakening to our true nature and inner wisdom. At some point we will even let go of our intentions, as yoga nidra is the ultimate practice of non-doing. If we are teachers of yoga nidra, every instruction to our students is offered as a blessing, with a sprinkling of love and the intention for them to awaken while sleeping. Once we understand that we are taking a journey toward something much more expansive and enlightening than a yoga nap, the practice becomes something we cherish, it's our secret portal to power. When we wake up from our practice, we are changed; we may have just tasted our true nature or the peace of *samadhi*. When we move back into our lives, the sweetness of that state travels with us, calling us back to the practice again and again. This is the promise of yoga nidra.

ORIENTATION OF THIS BOOK

Part one of *Radiant Rest* offers a brief overview of the origins of yoga nidra. It's important to take the time to learn about yoga nidra, its origins, and its benefits before you dive into the practice. This is part of the preparation for practicing and honors the tradition of yoga. Chapter 1 gives a short introduction to the history of yoga nidra, while chapter 2 looks at some of the science behind the practice.

Preparing to practice is the theme of part two. To begin, chapter 3 provides the context for my approach to yoga nidra. We will look at some of the obstacles to relaxation and talk about the factors that play a part in blocking us from our birthright of deep rest and spiritual awakening and how to navigate them.

We may not always have time for a long practice, but we can always find a few moments to turn inward each day. This is why chapter 4 describes the Householder's Flow, a practice for those who have busy lives—working in or outside the home, caring for children or elders—or responsibilities that don't allow for practicing at the same time, in the same place, and for the same duration every day. The chapter offers inspiration for ways to weave the thread of practice and awareness through your days and nights. Consider it a reframe for what it means to "practice" and a way to bring the sacred into daily life with devotion as opposed to discipline.

You don't need any fancy or expensive props to practice yoga nidra. But taking extra care in how, when, and where you practice will help you to feel supported, which is an essential part of the preparation. In chapter 5 you'll find ideas for setting up a yoga nidra nest and other insights for creating a nurturing practice environment.

Finally, part three presents practices and variations for you to try yourself. You'll get the most out of this book if you use the pre-practices, self-inquiry questions, and nature-amplification practices, along with the deep relaxation practices, to explore yoga nidra beyond the level of technique. My intention is to help you to experience deep relaxation, to inspire you to experiment with and do further study about the practice, and to prepare you to surrender and receive the grace of yoga nidra.

Here are a few of the essential elements you'll find in the practice chapters.

Pre-practices. Before each deep relaxation practice, you will find a number of pre-practices, including *bija* mantras (seed sounds), mantras, *sankalpa* (intention), asanas (physical postures), and pranayama (breathing exercises). I encourage you to experiment with these pre-practices to help support your yoga nidra practice. If you're not familiar with them already, guides to each practice are included in the appendix.

Bedtime and Wake-Up Rituals. Do you ever catch yourself in that moment just before you are about to fall asleep? Anyone who has woken themselves up just before nodding off in a lecture knows what that feels like. What if I told you there was magic in that moment? That transition is a little void. It is the void to which the journey of yoga nidra leads us. Of the many transitions throughout our day, the time between sleeping and waking is one of the most significant of all. In my own practice, setting an intention to practice while "sleeping" allowed me to experience a new life inside my dreams and to start and end my days in a container of purpose.

The transitions between the states are powerful portals to awakening. They take advantage of the hypnagogic (immediately before sleep) and hypno-pompic (immediately before waking) states. I've included mini bedtime and wake-up rituals to add to your day in every practice chapter.

Nature-Amplification Practices. Yoga nidra practice often asks us to con-jure up images of the sun, the moon, the stars, celestial light, and the cosmos. Yet the practices are usually taught inside a yoga studio or practiced inside at home. The original seers of yoga practiced in nature, and sages like Dattatreya considered twenty-four aspects of nature to be their gurus. Why not connect to nature, where these practices and states of consciousness were first realized, and begin to remember and revive our relationship with the natural world?

When we practice in nature, we can *feel* the earth supporting us, sense the vapors of the moon descending upon us, or if we are lucky, see the twinkling stars of the Milky Way. I live in the Santa Monica Mountains on traditional Tongva land where the "mountains meet the sea," and I teach annually in Big Sur, traditional Esselen land. These settings provided inspiration for restoring my connection to nature. I realized very quickly that renewing this connection was amplifying my yoga nidra practice and changing my life in unexpected ways. I was rewilding myself and allowing nature to heal me, awaken dormant wisdom, and transform my practice.

I no longer had to conjure up an image of a brilliant starlit sky; it was there, real. I could place each of those "tiny, blue, starlike points of light" in my body, in real time. When I went back to practicing in my house, my body remembered, and I returned to a vibration that felt very familiar. It felt like home. My practice was illuminated by the light and frequency of the elements and the natural world. My practice was becoming embodied with consistent practice and nature as a teacher. *Embodiment*, as I define it, is a sense of carrying the wisdom of the practice in your cells—you are in such a deep relationship with the practice that it becomes a part of you. For those of you who are teachers, this is a key component to being able to "transmit" a teaching to students.

Students have shared startling stories about how practicing in nature helped shift their practices and helped them move through fear of the unknown. Many were able to return to city life with an embodied remembrance of lying under the full moon or the stars, a memory that informed their practices for years. I offer these nature-amplification practices to honor nature as a teacher, to awaken your remembrance of your elemental nature, and to assist you in connecting to the wisdom of the earth.

Audio Recordings. Each of the deep relaxation practices is available as an audio recording to guide you. Visit www.Shambhala.com/RadiantRestPractices to access them. I recommend listening to the practices first and letting my voice guide you. Then read through the practices in the book. As you become more familiar with them, you'll be able to guide yourself. The conclusion has more ideas for self-guiding practices.

Questions for contemplation appear throughout the book. The practices of self-inquiry and self-study are a powerful part of the yogic path and lead to refined discernment and understanding. They have been invaluable tools in my own life and teaching. I recommend that you get a journal or notebook and commit time to freewriting your answers to the self-inquiry questions rather than just thinking about them. Don't worry about what you write or making the writing grammatically correct; just let it flow. You may be surprised what surfaces. If you resist the self-inquiry practices, consider what you might learn from that resistance. Sometimes your reaction to a question can lead you to deep truth if you're willing to look.

The end of the book offers an appendix with a brief overview of each kind of practice mentioned—from asanas to pranayama—as well as short descriptions of the different schools of yoga nidra. A glossary of terms is provided for easy reference, and the bibliography and recommended resources section will help you continue your studies if you wish to geek out and delve deeper.

HOW TO USE THIS BOOK

There are a few ways you can use this book. They are not mutually exclusive and are interchangeable. One day you might be exhausted and need a reset. Another day you might be working on something creative and want to tap into your intuition. Maybe you're brushing up on techniques to teach a class or workshop, or perhaps you're on a personal retreat with plenty of spaciousness to explore some of the practices in-depth. Maybe you are looking to touch the deepest levels of your being. Whatever you need from your practice, I recommend that you read the first chapters to understand the history of the practice and explore how to approach it. Then dive into the chapters that most resonate with your needs and intention for practice; go for what your life calls for in the moment.

If You Want to Experience Deep Relaxation. Flip to the practice section in part three that you feel you need most. Take time to answer the self-inquiry questions and listen to the recorded audio version of the practice. Give yourself plenty of time to transition out of the practice and get back into the rhythm of your day without feeling rushed. After exploring deep relaxation, you'll want to read the information in the first two chapters to understand more about what is happening during the practice.

If You Crave Rest and Ritual but Your Time Is Limited. Check out chapter 4 on the Householder's Flow. It shares small ways you can bring the sacred into your days when you don't have time for a longer practice.

If You're a Teacher. Go through the book systematically. Take time to do each practice regularly for a minimum of forty days. Use the nature-amplification practices to deepen your experiences and explore the elements within your own body. Choose one practice that you want to teach. Practice it consistently for forty days. Then begin to share it with a few students or another teacher in your community and get feedback before teaching a group. Seek out training with a teacher who can guide and mentor you.

If You're a Seeker. For the next year, work with this book as your guide and nature as an ally to help deepen your practice. Devote time to practice every day. Journal. Find friends who want to join the journey and compare notes with them. Read the recommended resources, check out the references that interest you, and don't be afraid to go down the rabbit hole. This is a lifelong practice.

Let your intuition guide you on this journey. There are no rules, just practice, so be curious and keep notes! However you choose to approach this practice, it will be revealing, relaxing, rejuvenating, and sometimes challenging. Yoga nidra is a healing salve for the world. I've been saying this repeatedly since I recorded my first yoga nidra practices in 2004. It is a practice that offers unconditional love and support while revealing that which has been hidden from view. It doesn't matter if you can get your leg behind your head. It doesn't matter if you believe in everything or nothing. You don't even need to "like" yoga. Everyone can receive its benefits and grace. The fact that the practice is done lying down makes it accessible to many people.

You must know this too. Maybe that's why you picked up this book. You have felt the magic or perhaps just heard about how powerful and inspiring it feels to wake up while you are sleeping. If we apply this healing salve to ourselves and openly receive and accept all the healing and awakening it brings, then just our presence in the world is healing. If we each share our love of this practice with just one of our beloveds, we can create movement toward the sacred self-care, self-love, and realization of Self that everyone on this planet deserves.

Thank you for joining me here. Thank you for your curiosity and courage. May these practices inspire, awaken, and nourish you. May they remind you of your inherent beauty, radiance, and power. May you connect to that place within you that is the doorway to truth and freedom. May you know that it is our shared birthright to be free, powerful, and radiant.

SELF-INQUIRY

1. What is your relationship with yoga nidra, deep relaxation, and rest?
2. What do you hope to get out of practicing with this book and audio recordings? Write the first few things that come to mind.

· PART 1 ·

The Depths of Yoga Nidra

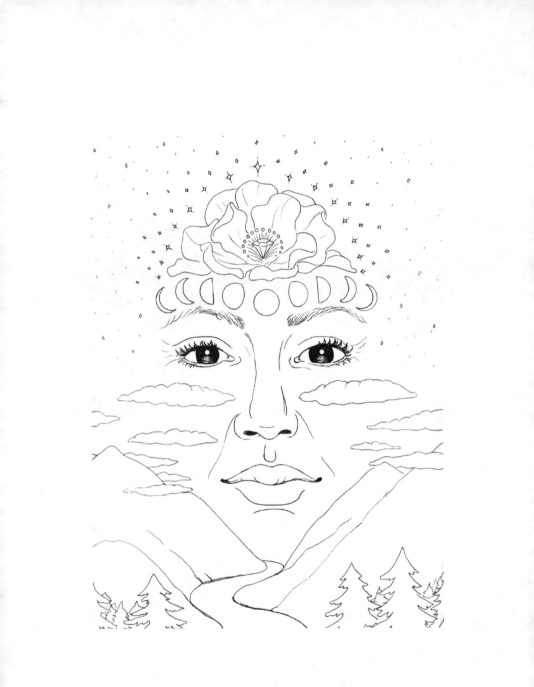

· 1 ·

The Mystery of Yoga Nidra

The Goddess

She is the Great Mother
The one who holds, nurtures, and supports
Unconditionally
Her body is the fertile soil of the earth
Her spine a flowing river
Her heart filled with a sea of liquid diamonds
Her eyes deep pools into an endless void
Her breath is rose-colored light filling you with love
Her face radiant like the full moon
She is waiting for you to surrender into her arms
So you might sleep while awake
Like the Divine child whose birthright is
deep rest, peace, and truth.

—Tracee Stanley

MANY INDIGENOUS CULTURES around the world have practices that explore the depths of the states of consciousness through meditation, sacred dreaming, and plant medicines. When the original seers of yoga first realized the state of consciousness associated with yoga nidra is not known. Yoga comes from the Sanskrit word *yuj*, which means "to connect, join, or balance."[1]

THE EIGHT LIMBS OF YOGA

Patanjali was an Indian philosopher who, somewhere between the second and fourth centuries, codified yoga into a systematic approach in writings known as the Yoga Sutras. Patanjali compiled 196 aphorisms, short teachings on the nature of yoga, that highlighted an eightfold path as the steps toward the realization of yoga. The eight limbs of yoga provide the opportunity for many lifetimes of study. The following list is simply a summary to introduce you to the concept or refresh your memory. The list of resources in the back of this book suggests other publications that offer more detail if you want to dive deeper into the Yoga Sutras.

- *Yamas*—restraints that help you transform negative tendencies. They include nonharming, truthfulness, nonstealing, restraint of power, and nongrasping.
- *Niyamas*—observances to help cultivate happiness and resiliency. They include cleanliness, contentment, austerity, self-study, and devotion to a Divine power.
- Asana—a steady and comfortable posture or seat.
- Pranayama—breath restraint to facilitate the direction and expansion of prana.
- *Pratyahara*—the withdrawal of the senses from external objects allowing to move inward and reassimilate into our true nature.
- Dharana—concentration achieved by fixing the mind in one place.
- Dhyana meditation—one-pointed focus of the mind. Meditation as a process.[2]
- Samadhi—a blissful union with the Divine. Meditation as the highest state.[3]

What new students find most surprising is that yoga nidra was often used as a synonym for samadhi, the goal of yoga, which is union with the Divine.[4]

This is where we get our first inkling that yoga nidra is much more than a technique and in fact a full system of yoga.

YOGA NIDRA TEACHINGS— PAST AND PRESENT

Yoga nidra is referred to in several texts, including the Devi Mahatmya (in the fifth to sixth century), Hatha Yoga Pradipika (in the fifteenth century), Yoga Taravali (around the fourteenth century), and the Mandala Brahmana Upanishad (date unknown), but none of them offer complete or detailed instructions on how to enter this state.[5]

The wisdom of yoga nidra is believed to have been passed down through oral tradition. This may be one reason why there is very little written detail about exactly how to do a practice that is accessible to Westerners and leads to the state of yoga nidra. The practice may have been reserved for students who were ready to receive deeper teachings. Powerful practices were often written in a way that only revealed themselves if the student had a certain level of understanding. Essential pieces were left out as a way both to protect the practices from those who might abuse them and to protect the students who were not ready for them.

HARM IN YOGA

As we begin to explore the recent history of yoga nidra, it is important to mention that like the history of other styles of yoga and spiritual traditions, yoga nidra is not without challenging elements and people who have used it to cause harm. There have been allegations of abuse against teachers who have popularized the practice and written books about it.

I want to pause to recognize this because I believe survivors. Power dynamics are real, and it is never okay for a teacher to harm students in any way— physically or emotionally. I also believe that this practice is a healing salve that allows us to connect to our inner wisdom and thus transcends any lineage or guru. As a student or practitioner of yoga nidra, you should feel empowered to ask questions of those sharing any practices with you, and to that end I have included information in the resources section that can help you if you have concerns.[6] I have found the second edition of Dr. Uma Dinsmore-Tuli's book *Yoni Shakti: A Woman's Guide to Power and Freedom through Yoga and Tantra* to have especially helpful information.

MODERN HISTORY OF YOGA NIDRA

Most of the prominent yoga nidra teachers in the past century gained wisdom by receiving teachings from their gurus, practicing for long periods of time, and learning from their experiences. They would then share what they had learned, and developed and refined techniques for their students.

Other teachers found themselves enveloped in the state of yoga nidra by Divine grace. They then developed systems of their own to try to enter the state intentionally again. Swami Veda Bharati, for example, accidentally discovered the practice of deep relaxation and the state of yoga nidra as a young boy in the mid-1900s. As a child prodigy, he went all over India giving lectures, and he was always exhausted and in poor health. He intuitively developed his own relaxation practice to overcome the effects of constant travel and fatigue. When he was thirty-six years old, he learned that the practice he'd been doing for so many years had a formal name and systematic technique called yoga nidra.[7]

Swami Satyananda, a prominent teacher in the second half of the twentieth century, was said to have experienced the state of yoga nidra and then constructed his own techniques from ancient texts that were not widely available at the time. Satyananda was charged with abuse; I mention him because the approach he shared has been influential in many styles of yoga nidra taught today.

Richard Miller, PhD, discovered the practice in 1970 in his first Hatha Yoga class and continued to return, eventually developing his own protocol known as iRest. He has done more than perhaps any modern school of yoga nidra to promote research testing of the practice and taking it to groups that would not otherwise have exposure to yoga practices, such as veterans struggling with post-traumatic stress disorder (PTSD).

Rod Stryker, another popular teacher today was one of my main teachers for well over a decade, was introduced to yoga nidra practices by his teacher, Mani Finger, decades ago. More recently he began to research and build on teachings he had been given in the Himalayan tradition. He created his own style and scripts for yoga nidra called Enlightened Sleep.

Amrit Desai learned about the technique from his teacher, Swami Kripalu, and began to share it in the 1980s. Desai developed more than one hundred scripts from the techniques he had learned. His daughter, Kamini, developed a systematic approach to make the teachings accessible, and together they created I AM Yoga Nidra (the Integrative Amrit Method of Yoga Nidra). Kamini Desai wrote a book, *Yoga Nidra: The Art of Transformational Sleep*, that details the practices and philosophy of her method.

In 2010, Uma Dinsmore-Tuli, PhD, and Nirlipta Tuli—cofounders of the Yoga Nidra Network—developed Total Yoga Nidra, an approach to sharing yoga nidra that incorporates various styles and is post-lineage, decolonized, creative, and spontaneously responsive.

No matter the technique, style, or tradition, the ability to powerfully transmit the practice as a teacher or prepare oneself to surrender into yoga nidra is bolstered by consistent practice and self-study. The power of deep rest, the Goddess, and the state of consciousness are the true teachers. It is said that one who "masters" yoga nidra no longer needs a technique to enter that state but can enter it "at will."

I mention teachers in the lineage of the Himalayan tradition because that is where I have primarily studied over the last twenty years. I have studied many types of yoga and tantra (the science of energy management), but the lineage of Himalayan masters and what I have learned through dedicated study are the foundation of my teaching style. I also incorporate what I have learned in other traditions in this book. I have the deepest gratitude for the generosity and wisdom of the teachers with whom I have studied. I am also grateful for being fortunate enough to have the means, access, and time to devote to thousands of hours of study. I have done my own research and lots of self-practice to deepen my exploration into what I have been taught. It is an important tantric concept that all of the teachings lead you back to your inner teacher, and the practice of yoga nidra is no different. No dogma is intended in these pages; there are many ways to practice, and they all lead to the same place. I invite you to be open, curious, and available for magic to happen in your practice.

THE MOTHER TEACHER

The lineage of the Himalayan tradition extends back thousands of years and is rooted in the wisdom of Patanjali's Yoga Sutras and tantra. Many of the teachings of this tradition were taught and popularized in the West by Swami Rama, a prolific author, a yogic scholar, and the founder of the Himalayan Institute in Honesdale, Pennsylvania. His life was not without controversy or documented allegations of abuse. I refer to him in this book, because his contribution to yoga nidra and the science of biofeedback was significant. In his book *Living with the Himalayan Masters*, Swami Rama described his journey through the Himalayas as he met and learned from great sages. One of these he referred to as "My Mother Teacher," or "Mataji." She was ninety-six at the time of their meeting (year unknown), and he described her as "a bag of bones wrapped inside shining skin. Her eyes were glowing like bowls of fire."[8]

He became intrigued by Mataji's solo nightly visits to the Kamakhaya temple in Assam from midnight to 3 a.m., when no one else was inside. He had heard that she did not sleep, so he secretly watched her practice, and his nightly spying confirmed it. After she angrily chased him away a few times, she finally gave him a blessing and accepted him as her student.

When Swami Rama asked Mataji about her lack of sleep, she scoffed and asked him if he knew about "sleepless sleep or yoga sleep." He had never heard of it. He then spent the next two and a half months learning from her during which time he took seventy pages of notes: "She explained to me the whole anatomy of sleep and asked me if I knew that mechanism in which a human being goes from the conscious state to the dreaming state and then to the deeper state of sleep. She started giving me accurate and systematic lessons. After that, I was able to understand the Mandukya Upanishad, which explains the three states of mind—waking, dreaming, sleeping—and the fourth state, *turiya*, which [Swami Rama] called 'the state beyond.'"

The technique of yoga nidra is a journey through the states of consciousness while remaining awake and aware. As we are guided through the practice, we are led closer and closer to the state of deep sleep and beyond to our true Self, or samadhi. But we also stay aware; we do not fall asleep to the beauty of our true nature. We are aware, and we are aware of awareness. This is what Mataji taught Swami Rama, and he later went on to write about these states of consciousness in great detail in his translation of the Mandukya Upanishad (*OM the Eternal Witness: Secrets of the Mandukya Upanishad*). For anyone interested in yoga nidra, it's essential to know about these states of consciousness and to develop an understanding of them through consistent practice and self-study. We will explore them in chapter 2.

It is also important to recognize a woman's role in the lineage of the Himalayan masters, as it relates to transmission of the practice of "sleepless sleep." Yoga nidra connects us to the universal energy of the Mother, which includes the feminine qualities of nurturing, support, rejuvenation, receptivity, and surrender. If we can remember this great Mother Teacher, Mataji, or the energy of the Universal Mother at the beginning of our yoga nidra practice, we honor a lineage of teachers, including our own ancestral mothers even if we do not know their names.

THE GODDESS YOGA NIDRA

Another feminine power in this practice is the Goddess Yoga Nidra. I had been practicing the technique for many years before I heard Yoga Nidra referred to as a Goddess. Some of the earliest known uses of the term refer not to a specific yoga practice, as we often think of it today, but to the Divine Mother, the personification of the feminine creative power. The scientist and religious studies teacher Sreedevi Bringi first introduced me to this teaching in a workshop through the beautiful Devi Suktam, a hymn praising the Divine Mother and her many powers that uphold the universe. One of the verses says, *Ya Devi sarva bhuteshu Nidra-rupena samsthitha / Namastasye Namastasye Namastasye Namo Namaha.* It can be translated as "the Goddess expresses herself in the form of Sleep. The Sleeping state in you is a form of the Mother Divine. As sleep, She is present in every being."[9]

One version of the story of the Goddess describes how Brahma, the Creator, was sitting on a lotus growing out of the navel of Vishnu, the Preserver and Protector. Vishnu was in a deep, dreamless sleep, a cosmic yoga nidra in the transition between the cycles of creation and destruction. Meanwhile Brahma was attacked by two demons. Brahma desperately needed help, but Vishnu was in such a deep sleep, filled with inertia, that he wasn't responsive to Brahma's cries. No matter what Brahma did, he could not wake Vishnu. So he decided that he needed to call on the Goddess Yoga Nidra, who had taken her seat within Vishnu to support his deep, meditative sleep. To call on Yoga Nidra, Brahma began to sing her praises. He extolled her virtues of cooling, nurturing, and moonlike qualities over and over, until she became manifest. She answered Brahma's prayers, brought Vishnu out of his cosmic sleep, asked him to slay the two demons, and used her powers to confuse the minds of the demons so Vishnu could destroy them. In this story, the Goddess's power is so supreme that even the most powerful gods must depend on her grace.[10]

Yes, it's true—we are all powerless without the grace of sleep. I'll be sharing the hymn and a practice that will connect you to the moonlike quality of yoga nidra later in the book.

"These early references to the term *yoganidra* are not defining a practice or a technique in a system of yoga but are describing a god's transcendental sleep and the goddess' manifestation as sleep," Jason Birch and Jacqueline Hargreaves wrote in their brilliant essay "Yoganidrā: An Understanding of the History and Context."[11]

If you're inspired by the beauty and power of this story, you can begin to layer your practice with devotion to the nurturing and healing force of the Divine Mother. Imagine framing your yoga nidra practice as a prayer or petition to receive the grace of deep conscious sleep—a sleep that gives you deep rest but also awakens you to the most powerful parts of yourself. The journey of this practice takes place on a few different levels, as we will discuss in the next chapter, and exploring them helps us to understand the kind of yogic sleep that is possible with yoga nidra.

YOUR OWN YOGA NIDRA JOURNEY

Please remember that there is immense value in researching various schools, approaches, and teachers. I encourage you to embark on your own exploration in practice, keep a yoga nidra journal, and connect with others who are also dedicated to exploring the practice in depth. "Knowledge does not flow from authority or information," as Neil deGrasse Tyson said.[12] True knowledge flows from our inner wisdom. I find that people who are devoted to deeply knowing yoga nidra as a state consider themselves "forever students" as opposed to just trying to quickly "get it" or adding another tool to their yoga tool kit to make themselves stand out as teachers.

The gifts of yoga nidra are endless, and this is a lifelong practice.

· 2 ·

The Journey through Consciousness

REMEMBER THE STORY of Yoga Nidra as a mythical goddess that possesses supreme nurturing qualities and can bestow a dreamless, cosmic sleep, as we explore the depths of this sleep further. This chapter examines some of the philosophical concepts that inform the technique of yoga nidra as the means to reach samadhi, as well as how science seems to support these ideas. Ever since the electroencephalogram (EEG) was invented in the 1920s to look at the pulses of electrical activity in the brain (brain waves), researchers have studied what happens in our brains when our bodies sleep. The rishis and rishikas had been observing the stages of consciousness, the body, and sleep for centuries longer, as described in ancient texts such as the Mandukya Upanishad. Both brain waves and the stages of sleep seem to overlay the stages of consciousness described in the ancient texts.

Yoga nidra is a yoga of dissolution, or *laya* yoga. The practice moves our awareness from the most gross aspect of ourselves—the physical body—into awareness of the subtle body and eventually into a sense of dissolving into spaciousness. This is a journey through energetic sheaths (*koshas*) that are said to cover the light of the soul.

This chapter summarizes both the ancient teachings and Western science. I've suggested more detailed resources here and in the back of the book in case you want to go down the rabbit hole of one or all of these teachings.

THE SWAMI AND THE EEG

Just as scientific researchers have studied the physical impact of mindfulness meditation, they have also studied the impact of deep meditative states, including yoga nidra. Some of the first research in this area was conducted in the summer of 1970 by Elmer Green, PhD, a scientist at the Menninger Institute in Topeka, Kansas, who believed that the mind could play a big part in preventing and curing disease. His research explored whether "people can learn to voluntarily control physiologic functions that are normally involuntary," such as someone having no measurable pain or bleeding when the skin is pierced by a thick needle.[1]

Dr. Green and his wife and colleague, Alyce Green, had heard about a few people who claimed to have extraordinary powers in psychophysiological self-regulation, and they wanted to study these individuals to see what was really happening. Swami Rama, for one, claimed that he could stop his heart and regulate his blood pressure. Dr. Green invited the swami to participate in a series of experiments that Green hoped would give new understanding of the capacity of the human mind.

The Greens hooked the swami up to various electromagnetic machines to measure his "voluntary control of internal states." The success of these experiments would lie in the swami's ability not only to turn off internal states but also to turn them back on. Over the course of two summers, Swami Rama succeeded at demonstrating his ability to control blood flow in his hand; stop his heart for ten seconds; move a needle by chanting a mantra (telekinesis); and produce theta brain waves, as measured by EEG, that he called "stilling the conscious and bringing forward the unconscious."

By intentionally creating specific brain wave patterns, Swami Rama put himself into various states of consciousness. Training his body to respond to commands and regulate body functions over which we normally have no control (autogenic programming) and using visualization to tell his body what to do, he achieved a state of conscious relaxation. Dr. Green recounts in his writing "Biofeedback and Yoga,"[2] "He called this state 'yogic sleep' and said it was better than normal sleep."[3] Swami Rama could enter this state at will "producing an EEG record much like deepest sleep with 40 percent delta waves."[4]

These demonstrations led them to the banks of the Ganges River in India to study other yogis who had similar *siddhis* (powers) and informed the development of clinical biofeedback, which the Greens originated and to which they devoted their lives.

YOUR BRAIN WAVES

Brain waves are oscillating electrical charges in the brain, and they change according to what we are doing and feeling. The following sections describe the five widely recognized types of brain waves, from fastest to slowest. Although one brain wave state may predominate at any given time, depending on the activity level of the individual, the remaining states are present at all times.[5]

Gamma

Science is still learning about gamma waves. We know they are the fastest measurable brain waves and occur during peak events or moments of heightened perception—such as out-of-body experiences. Gamma activity is involved in attention, working memory, and long-term memory processes and in psychiatric disorders such as schizophrenia, hallucination, Alzheimer's disease, and epilepsy. These brain waves had not yet been discovered at the time of the Greens' experiments with the yogis.[6]

Beta

With beta brain waves, our awareness is external, concerned with the outside world. We are alert, attentive, and engaged. We may experience three types:

LO BETA—while reading a book

BETA—while attending a lecture or solving a problem

HI BETA—in a state of high anxiety or excitement

Alpha

Alpha waves happen when our eyes are closed, and our attention is directed internally, such as during yoga, meditation, and mindful presence. This is where we first begin to draw the five senses inward, known in yogic philosophy as *pratyahara* (withdrawal of the senses).

Theta

Theta waves are our gateway to learning, memory, and intuition. The theta state exists during deep relaxation, deep meditation, daydreaming, and dreaming during sleep.

Delta

Delta waves indicate that external awareness has been suspended and are seen in someone who is in a dreamless state of sleep, during a drug-induced coma, or under general anesthesia. Delta waves allow for healing and rejuvenation. They are necessary for good sleep that rejuvenates the body, revitalizes the brain, and strengthens the immune system. These were the brain waves that Swami Rama produced at will. Dean Radin, PhD, of the Institute of Noetic Sciences in Petaluma, California, told me that during experiments decades later Swami Veda Bharati also produced delta brain waves while fully conscious. Radin was having a casual conversation with Swami Veda while the swami was being hooked up to an EEG monitor, and as they continued to talk, the technician alerted them that Swami Veda was already in delta state. This was a surprise to both men and perhaps was an indication of Swami Veda's mastery of the state of yoga nidra.

STAGES OF SLEEP

Our stages of sleep can also be measured by EEG, and they're closely connected to our brain waves. The stages of sleep are known as REM and non-REM (NREM) stages 1, 2, 3, and 4. As we sleep, we oscillate between the stages every ninety minutes or so. Matthew Walker, PhD, illustrates this flip-flop between stages in his book, *Why We Sleep*.[7] The deepest quality of sleep is found in the NREM stages when the brain wave states move between theta and delta.[8]

The deepest stage of yoga nidra is associated with brain activity that indicates the subject should be sleeping, but EEG readings suggest that the person isn't actually asleep and has a level of conscious awareness. People practicing yoga nidra tend to produce theta and delta brain waves and still remain conscious. A 1999 study in Copenhagen, in which yoga nidra practitioners' brain activity was monitored during a positron-emission tomography (PET) scan, found something interesting:

> The measurements of the brain's activity (EEG) indicated that the subjects were in a deeply relaxed state, similar to that of sleep, during the whole yoga nidra. The theta activity rose significantly (11%) on all the twenty-one electrodes. The reduction of the alpha activity (2% NS) was insignificant, showing that this meditative state is altogether different from that of the sleeping state and comprises conscious awareness. Furthermore, the state was constant and evenly distributed over the entire brain for the forty-five minutes the relaxation lasted.[9]

Not only did they produce brain waves, but the people being studied also traveled through the states of consciousness represented by the sound and syllable AUM.

THE THREE STATES OF CONSCIOUSNESS AND THE FOURTH STATE

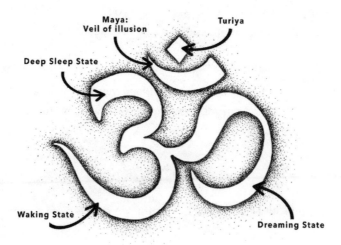

The states of consciousness and the power of the sound and syllable of AUM are explained in the twelve verses of the Mandukya Upanishad. It offers us a window to the levels of consciousness as steps toward enlightenment. The practice of yoga nidra asks us to bring awareness to each of the four states of consciousness and the transitions between them while remaining in relaxed awareness.

Take a moment to consider each of the three states of consciousness and "the fourth" with the self-inquiry questions that follow.

Waking (*Vaishvanara*)

In this state, the consciousness is directed to the external and perceived through the instruments of perception, such as the ears, eyes, nose, skin, and so on. We are focused on our physical body and the outer world.[10]

SELF-INQUIRY

1. What are you attached to in the external world? What causes you pleasure, and what causes you pain?
2. What does external success mean to you?
3. How can you be more conscious of your actions?

Dreaming (*Taijasa*)

Here, the consciousness is turned inward, and we become aware of mental impressions. We do not control these impressions. We have moved from the external to the internal.

SELF-INQUIRY

1. Is it difficult to turn your mind off from concerns of the outer world?
2. Do your dreams ever feel more real than your waking life?
3. How often do you daydream?
4. What do you daydream about most often? Is there a common theme?

Deep Sleep (*Prajna*)

At this stage, dreaming ends, and the mind quiets. We fall into darkness. We are aware of this only after we awaken, feeling of having been somewhere profound but being unable to remember it. This state of consciousness is the portal to the knowledge of the waking and dreaming states.

SELF-INQUIRY

1. How do you feel after you have awoken from a deep sleep?
2. How do you know that you have slept deeply? What essence

or quality do you bring back to the waking state from deep sleep?

The Fourth (*Turiya*)

This experience is beyond description. *Turiya* is the awareness behind all the other states; it is the unknown Knower. It is said that when we experience turiya, we have achieved *nirvikalpa samadhi*, experiencing "no mind"; only peace, infinite bliss, and pure consciousness remain. Turiya is the realization of the one true self, and in some traditions, there are seven stages of turiya.[11] When we experience the state of yoga nidra, we have entered the portal to turiya.

> That which is threading through these three states and even surpasses the sense "I am" is what you are. This is the fourth state Turiya.[12]
>
> —*Sri Ramanananda*

> Waking, dreaming, and deep sleep states are states where duality is experienced, for the experiencer is different from the experience. But the fourth state, Turiya, is a nondualistic state which is compared to the silence into which one is [led] by Om.[13]
>
> —*Swami Rama*

SELF-INQUIRY

1. What is the most profound experience you have had during or after yoga nidra or deep relaxation practice?
2. What is your personal definition of spiritual freedom? Notice where you feel restricted or resistant to the idea or feeling of freedom. Describe this resistance with words, poetry, or art.
3. What do you imagine freedom looks like for all beings on this earth?

· Pranava Practice ·

[5–30 minutes]

Pranava (cosmic sound) relates to meditating on the mantra AUM. It is said that AUM is a container for the Divine; in other words, it is a covering or sheath, and by invoking AUM, we invoke the Divine. All three states of consciousness and the fourth state are reflected in the sound and syllable of AUM. Repeating this sound is also a way to attune ourselves to our true nature, bridging the individual and the universal. After chanting AUM, allow for silence, letting yourself feel the vibration in the silence. Try the following practice:

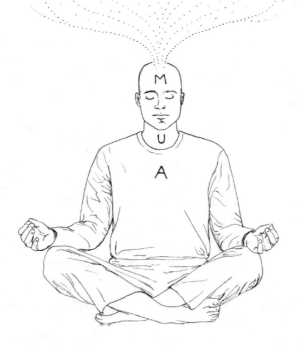

STAGE 1

Sit in a comfortable position on a chair or cross-legged on the floor.

Begin to chant the mantra AUM, pronouncing each syllable. Allow yourself to move into a two-pronged awareness. You are aware that you are chanting AUM. And you are aware of that part of you that is watching and hearing you chant AUM. (1 minute)

A (*ah*): As you chant this sound, contemplate the waking state. What does it feel like to be awake, eyes open and taking in the world?

U (*uu*): As you chant this sound, contemplate the dreaming state. Let yourself return to the space of whatever dreams you remember from the night before. Feel as though you are there in the dream.

M (*mm*): As you chant this sound, contemplate the deep sleep state, and feel as though you are moving deeper inward and dissolving into spaciousness.

STAGE 2

As you chant each syllable, let your attention move downward to the corresponding area:

A: the third eye
U: the throat center
M: the heart center
Silence: deeper into the spaciousness of the heart (2 minutes)

STAGE 3

As you chant each syllable, let your attention move upward to the corresponding area:

A: the heart center
U: the throat center

M: the third eye

Silence: into the space above the head (2 minutes)

Remember that part of you that was there when the world was
created. (1 minute)

Remember the ancient part of you that remembers the sound of
AUM. Feel the vibration in every cell of your body. (2 minutes)

When you complete the practice, make notes about your experience. What did you feel, sense, or see? Perhaps you began to sense that you are more than this physical body, more than gross matter. Maybe you felt the space inside and outside of your body full of vibration. If you did, you might be tuning in to subtle energy. You'll learn more about the subtle body soon.

PUTTING IT TOGETHER: SLEEP STATES, STATES OF CONSCIOUSNESS, AND BRAIN WAVES

One research article defined yoga nidra as "a state where the practitioner demonstrates the symptoms of deep non-REM sleep, including delta brainwaves, while simultaneously remaining fully conscious." This same research indicated that yoga nidra has four levels of practice that move us through stages:

1. During deep relaxation, alpha waves move into theta waves as the practice deepens.
2. During deeper practice, when the brain displays creativity or problem solving, theta waves verge on delta waves.
3. When the transition to the state of yoga nidra takes place, theta waves are followed by delta waves as the student drops into non-REM sleep but remains aware of their surroundings.
4. Once the other three levels have been mastered, the student's mind can remain in the two states of deep sleep and conscious awareness simultaneously.

"When Levels 3 and 4 are mastered one may gradually transition into turiya, during which yoga nidra and turiya (the fourth) become indistinguishable," and the student will be in a place of *nirvikalpa*, or "no thought." This is also known as the stage of samadhi, the final goal of yoga. This is where the mind merges into the heart, and prana (vital life force) returns to its source.[14]

Ramana Maharshi described turiya and nirvikalpa this way:

> Turiya is the mind in quiescence and aware of Self. There is the aware-ness that the mind has merged in its source. Whether the senses are active or inactive is immaterial. In nirvikalpa samadhi the senses are inactive. To know implies the subject and object. To be aware means to be thought-free.[15]

It is important to remember that when we have mastered yoga nidra (the non-REM, or delta, state), we can enter it at will, with no technique needed. In this process, we move from the most gross and material plane of existence to the most subtle.

This is why we need a general knowledge of what the subtle body (koshas) comprises.

THE KOSHAS: A JOURNEY THROUGH YOUR SPIRITUAL ANATOMY

The koshas are layers of consciousness that move from the gross to the subtle and cover the light of the soul, not to be confused with the *states* of consciousness. If you cut the body open, you will not see these coverings, because they are part of the energetic subtle anatomy as opposed to the physical anatomy. The layers are described in the Taittiriya Upanishad, an essential teaching from Vedanta that helps us to understand how yoga and the path toward samadhi works.

If you think of the coverings as Russian nesting dolls, you can imagine a brilliant light that burns brightly inside the smallest doll. However, as each doll is placed inside a larger doll, over time the light in the innermost doll is forgotten. If you see the entire set of dolls put together, from the outside, you see only one doll—the outer shell. It's easy to forget that you are so much more than just what you see, that you are the light and that light is radiance, truth, and beauty.

Some teachings say that part of your spiritual journey is to transcend the koshas, moving away from identification with the physical (that which is always decaying and dying) and toward tasting the eternal (your radiance).

There are five koshas:

Annamaya kosha: the food body
Pranamaya kosha: the energy body
Manomaya kosha: the mental body
Vijnanamaya kosha: the wisdom body
Anandamaya kosha: the bliss body

Let's take a closer look at each of them.

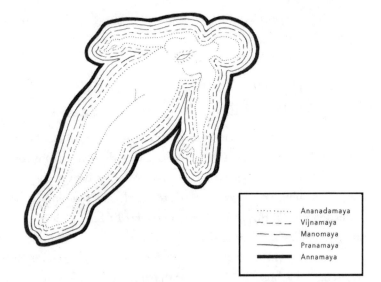

··········	Ananadamaya
– – – –	Vijnamaya
— — —	Manomaya
————	Pranamaya
▬▬▬	Annamaya

Annamaya Kosha: The Food Body

Over time your yoga journey opens a window to understanding the world of the subtle. You may have come to the yoga mat to get in shape, become more flexible, get a "yoga butt" (no judgment), or cure some aches and pains. Like most of us, you have probably been conditioned to understand that "you are what you eat," that you are the physical body, the thing you see in the mirror. That is who you know as "me." When we feel that the physical body is who and what we are, we are identifying with the outmost shell of our subtle anatomy—annamaya kosha, often translated as the "food body."

Pranamaya Kosha: The Energy Body

At the start of your yoga journey, you should be introduced to pranayama and breathing exercises. You may begin to feel energy moving in your body as heat, a tingling sensation, or involuntary jerks or twitches. As you learn techniques like Prana Dharana, you may find that you can direct this energy with the power of your mind, even when you are completely still. You might chant mantras and feel that you are coming alive in a new way; the space both inside and around your body feels pregnant with vibration. You may develop a new awareness that you must be more than just your physical body.

You—and everything else—are made of energy, and that energy is always changing. Your body is animated by an unseen force. There is a vital life force that is the source of life and is different than the breath. That vital life force is called *prana*; the breath is its primary vehicle, and food is its delivery system.[16] Every form of physical exercise, asana, or pranayama in which you engage affects your prana. With the help of skilled teachers, you can learn how to create alchemy and sequence your practices for specific effects and outcomes. As you become more sensitive to prana, you become more aware of pranamaya kosha, the energy body.

Manomaya Kosha: The Mental Body

As you continue down the road of yoga practice, you may begin to notice the everyday barrage of constant thoughts, amazed that you could be thinking so much *all the time*. Thoughts are like reverberations of all our life experiences; they become the coloring of habits and when those habits are concretized, they form our personality and worldview. When you practice yoga, especially some of the quieter practices such as yin, restorative, meditation, and yoga nidra, you may start to observe your mind and how it is always changing. Breathing techniques help to calm the mind and also give a reflection into the quality of mind.

Self-inquiry practices can help you become aware of your thoughts and how they are shaping your life. Inquiring into the source of your beliefs allows you to discover how the past may be holding you prisoner. The more you move, breathe, meditate, and study yourself, the less you are a prisoner of your thoughts and more like an observer who knows the prison door is not really locked. If you can just turn your face in the other direction, you might see the doorway to freedom. Your daily practice becomes a way of reminding yourself that there is a door, and you begin to inch your way toward it. You become aware that you have a choice in which direction are you turning—toward the old repeating thoughts and patterns that are based on the past or toward the discernment that is available in the present moment. When we begin to observe the functions of the mind as separate from who we really are, we have awareness of the manomaya kosha, or the mental body.

Vijnanamaya Kosha: The Wisdom Body

Who hasn't been on the yoga mat or meditation cushion, having a long run, or walking in nature and had an epiphany? It is a knowing that seems to descend out of nowhere. One of the translations of *vijnanamaya* is "to suddenly come into view." It may be such a profound visceral feeling of knowing or understanding that you don't question it. You feel it in every cell of your body. This is a higher level of consciousness that resides in the intuitive, or wisdom, body. Truth has a frequency, and it takes time to cultivate the trust within yourself to eliminate the doubt and fear that comes with following your inner voice. When you recognize truth, it has a vibration. The more you practice, the more you attune yourself to that vibration. It is here that you may begin to sense that there is something constant and powerful that resides within you that is not subject to change.

Before you get to this place of knowing, you have to remove a stain that stands in your way of truth, and that is the stain of your beliefs, residue of the manomaya kosha. These beliefs can be tricky; they are like a loop of thoughts in which they reinforce each other. Dismantling your beliefs may feel like you are dissolving—and part of you will. It's work. By doing practices that remind you of something greater than yourself, by doing self-inquiry, and by being with others who are interested in doing deeper work, you can begin to cultivate discernment to tell the difference between your beliefs and true wisdom. Our practice then becomes a constant reminder to turn toward the light of discernment.

Anandamaya Kosha: The Bliss Body

Remember your first blissful Savasana or meditation? The one that kept you coming back to yoga? It's possible that you tasted the sweetness of anandamaya kosha, or bliss body. And in that bliss, you may have had a feeling that none of what you have identified with in your whole life is real. Your body, your thoughts, your beliefs, your intellect; they're not the real you. You feel for a split second that you are so much more. Expansive, radiant, and free. *You* are everything and everywhere. You are limitless and boundless. If you taste that even for a second, you will never be the same again. You will *always* know who and what you truly are.

The steps toward yoga nidra help us to move toward the ethereal, beyond space and time, to touch our eternal radiance. Most schools of yoga nidra acknowledge a progression of steps that can move us through the koshas. Yoga nidra as a technique is a journey from the gross to the subtle that leads to the state of consciousness that can only be accessed in the depths of spacious silence and grace. Although the journey through the koshas is presented as linear, it is common to move between states of consciousness or have varied experiences such as noticing your own snoring, having flashes of visual images, being aware of energy moving and sounds emerging, and observing physical discomfort or emotions arising. Once you begin to explore them in practice, your understanding of the koshas will deepen.

THE SPACE BETWEEN

Your yoga nidra teacher may have asked you to remain "awake and aware" during your practice. As we are guided through the states of consciousness and stages of sleep, we need to stay aware. Aware to the transitions, especially the moments when we feel the body becoming heavy, the breath is shallower, and we begin to fall into a liminal dreamy space known as the hypnagogic state. Verse 75 of Swami Lakshmanjoo's translation of the Vijnana Bhairava Tantra says, "By entering that state that precedes sleep where the awareness of the outer world has faded the mind is absorbed in the threshold state which the supreme goddess illumines."[17] Our practice allows us to move into a more effortless awareness, as opposed to waiting for something to happen or looking for an experience.

In *Why We Sleep*, Matthew Walker tells the story of Thomas Edison, who was also a dedicated napper.[18] According to legend, the inventor would nap in a chair holding three steel ball bearings and with a metal plate directly underneath him on the floor. The moment he drifted off, the balls would fall out of his hand and onto the plate, waking him up. He would immediately get up and write down all his creative ideas; he called this his "genius gap." Albert Einstein napped with a metal spoon in his hand and a metal plate on the floor. Einstein's theory of relativity is said to have come to him during a dream. One can only wonder if Edison and Einstein had discovered the power of yogic sleep and the transition between states, using it as a portal to amplify creativity and genius.

We all hold our own unique genius, and staying awake during the transitions between the states of consciousness may hold the key to realizing our superpowers.

The neuroscientist and artist Nkechi Njaka described the transition to me this way: "Hypnagogia is the liminal space that exists between wakefulness and sleep—beginning at the onset, when the mind is first impacted by sleepiness, and concluding when the mind finally loses consciousness. This transitional phase lasts only a few minutes and includes lucid thought, lucid dreaming, and hallucinations. The experience of this space is far less immersive than a dream experienced in REM sleep and has often been a space artists rely on to amplify their creative expression."[19] Our practice helps us to recognize these transitions and stay awake and aware during them as opposed to blacking out.

The transition is also a gateway to turiya. Swami Lakshmanjoo described this as a "gap" in *Kashmir Shaivism: The Secret Supreme*: "This gap is a junction between the waking state and the dreaming state. There is also a junction between the dreaming state and dreamless sound sleep and there is a junction between sound sleep and the waking state. This junction is only a gate, the entrance to turiya. . . . This junction is known to be the start of turiya. In entering this junction, the aspirant enters into another world. It is not wakefulness, nor is it the dreaming state, nor is it sound sleep, but a fourth world."[20] Lakshmanjoo gives us further direction on how to enter this state; we must concentrate on the centers of the heart, but he does not mention how—and he refers to "centers" meaning more than one place at the heart. This is one of those teachings that were held secret by lineages and would likely have been taught to students one on one or in very small groups. The swami's writing also suggests that if we practice this when we go to bed, we will fall into a deep, dreamless sleep. All the more reason to practice the bedtime rituals in this book!

Before you get started with these rituals, I suggest you try a few days of practice with the mental alarm clock. The practice of setting a mental alarm clock is also a great way to introduce a helpful bedtime practice that allows you to explore that part of yourself that is always awake. Since I learned this practice more than twenty years ago, I have very rarely used an alarm clock.

SETTING YOUR MENTAL ALARM CLOCK

Before going to sleep, note the time. Close your eyes and visualize the time as it would appear on an analog clock face. See the hands of the clock begin to move until they arrive at the time when you would like to get up. Pause as you see the hands of the clock at that time and repeat silently to yourself, *I will wake up at _____ o'clock and then go to sleep.* The key to this practice is to let go. It's not a competition or something to get perfect. Go into this one with a sense of curiosity so you are not up all night checking the clock!

THE SACRED PORTALS

So far we have discussed ideas like "the mind merges into the heart" and that we must "concentrate on the centers of the heart." These instructions point us to one of the secrets to entering the state of yoga nidra. We now find ourselves looking at the four limbs of yoga, pratyahara (withdrawal of the senses) serves as a link between pranayama and dharana.[21] We move from concentration (dharana) toward one-pointedness of the mind in meditation (dhyana) and perhaps to the point where we merge with and realize the radiant, luminous, and infinite Self (samadhi).

Four places of concentration, or portals, have the power to lead you toward transcendental consciousness:

1. The spot between the eyebrows (*bhrumadhya*): The center is said to be the center of waking.
2. The hollow pit of the throat (*kaṇṭha kupa*): Many traditions consider this the center of dreaming. Practices of lucid and sacred dreaming often focus on the throat.
3. The heart (*hridaya*)[22]: Some traditions pay special attention to the heart center as a place of concentration. In fact, their followers will say that you are not practicing yoga nidra "properly" unless

you rest at the heart center. Initiatory meditation practices on the heart are said to allow one to know what is unknown and to amplify the powers of self-healing.

4. The womb: The womb space has long been considered a place of the great void, transition, creativity, and fertility. It is symbolic of the Great Mother and is said to contain the entire universe. There is also an energetic connection between the womb and the heart. The heart-womb meridian runs like a "river of light" between the heart and the womb.[23] This practice involves bringing awareness to the pelvic region, and it's one that anyone can explore—no matter how you identify your gender and even if you have had a hysterectomy. Students have reported feeling this connection with the heart prior to knowing it existed. This is an example of letting the practice teach you.

It has been my experience that each portal has its own unique gifts that should be explored, and certain teachings say that the first three of these portals lead to samadhi. Do your own experimentation by resting awareness in each one after deep relaxation, making notes and coming to your own conclusions through your own experience. If you are a teacher of yoga nidra, such experimentation is essential. We'll talk more about this in later chapters, where you will learn practices that can help you to tap into clarity, knowing, and a deep trust that you are always supported. But how does that work?

SUPERPOWERS ACTIVATE

Waves of inspiration and creativity can come to us like "downloads," when we suddenly feel plugged into something greater than ourselves. These downloads can occur in moments of deep presence or in being awake and aware to a transition from one state of being to another just like Edison. When we are tapped into universal consciousness, we can connect with an infinite source of wisdom. This can happen while spending time in nature or during long periods of silence, dreams, meditation, yoga nidra, running, or dancing; the opportunities are endless as long as you are present.

The Yoga Sutras refer to eight mystical powers that come from practice as siddhis, or accomplishments. They include control over the elements and the ability to make yourself tiny or enormous, to name two. It sounds like fun, but these powers are obstacles to the goal of yoga. You don't want to become attached to these newfound powers, because one of the most important aspects of the yogic path is detachment; the other is practice. These siddhis aren't talked about much in yoga and meditation trainings, but they should be. We can't ignore that once we begin to do any kind of meditation or yoga nidra consistently, we will start to notice some interesting phenomena. In a 2018 research study on advanced meditators and mystical experiences, scientists were able to explore this idea:

> Advanced meditators have demonstrated at least twelve perceptual capacities that scientists once dismissed as impossible. These capacities include, for example, lucid dreaming, lucid nondream sleep, and heightened perceptual speed and sensitivity. What further capacities await recognition? Over half of the meditators in our sample reported experiencing clairvoyance or telepathy (perceiving information that could not have been known to them by any known physical means, but later turned out to be true) at least once. Not only that, but the majority also found the experience "somewhat pleasant" and "quite meaningful or important.[24]

If we remember that our yoga nidra practice is a simultaneous journey through the koshas, the states of consciousness, and the brain wave states, it is no wonder that people describe the practice as everything from "cosmic" and "out of this world" to "a trip to the void." Our practice holds magic. As we discussed earlier, staying awake and aware during transitions leads us to a powerful portal into a cosmic realm. It's important to proceed with reverence for the practice and to seek out the support of a qualified teacher or therapist if needed.

So, what does it mean to have a superpower in our everyday lives? It means we have the unwavering courage to lean into and trust the inner knowing and clarity that arises from practice. When we have that awakened clarity, we rise in power with laser-like focus and the energy to explore our passions and inspirations. Without concern for what other people believe we are capable of, we know that we are supported by something much greater than ourselves.

BASIC PRACTICE STEPS

The many schools of yoga nidra all have progressive steps that help to lead the practitioner from awareness of the gross to the subtle and eventually to rest in awareness, presence, and the deepest states of relaxation. Various teachers and traditions have their own specific order to, protocols for, and additions to or subtractions from this list according to their own lineage experience, the desired outcome for the practice, and the groups they are teaching.

This section gives a general outline of the steps commonly used and the order in which they are often taught; however, it is best to respond to your current needs or the needs of the student by being present to what arises and using the various tools to address those needs. This is why having an embodied understanding of the practice is especially important for teachers.

Notice how we gradually move from focusing on the physical body to more subtle levels of presence, stillness, and spaciousness. It's important to remember that the experience isn't always linear, so it's good to stay open and receptive.

PRE-PRACTICE. Gentle movements, mantras, or breathing practices to prepare the body to release tension and surrender. The mind is directed inward, and an attitude of gratitude for the practice is cultivated. Take a moment to honor the practice and remember why you are practicing.

RELAXED AND SUPPORTED POSTURE. Savasana, side-lying poses, restorative poses, or any other posture in which the body can feel fully supported. Add as many props as you need—don't skimp. This relates to the third limb of yoga, asana, and cultivating a "seat" that is steady yet effortless.

DIAPHRAGMATIC BREATHING. One of the essential and often overlooked part of practice is establishing effortless breathing. We can begin by bringing attention to the navel area moving up and down with each inhalation and exhalation. With practice, we can cultivate a diaphragmatic breath that is silent, effortless, smooth, deep, even, and continuous.[25] This awareness of the breath can activate the body's rest-and-digest state. Pranayama, the fourth limb of yoga, is addressed here as the awareness of prana expands, and the mind moves toward stability.

PRATYAHARA. As we withdraw our awareness of the external stimuli by pulling our senses inward, the mind begins to still. This is the most important step in yoga nidra. It is the process of gradual dissolution. The awareness of sounds, sight, taste, touch, and smells are withdrawn, and our pull toward them is loosened. The teachings say that as a tortoise withdraws their limbs with ease, so one should withdraw the senses together with the mind.[26] It is pratyahara that moves us toward spiritual liberation and the bridge that links the limbs of yoga.

SANKALPA. The acknowledgment of a resolve, intention, or affirmation. Though sankalpa or affirmations are often suggested, they are not always used or necessary. As we move into deeper experiences of the state of yoga nidra, sankalpa is released, and we move into "non-doing."

SYSTEMATIC RELAXATION OF THE BODY. Relaxation of parts of the body. Awareness of breath, feeling that the body is breathing you, letting go of effort and "doing." It is here that we become aware that there is an outside force that compels us to breathe, and we surrender to that involuntary action of breathing.

VISUALIZATION. The formation of and focus on a mental image of a specific thing, points of light, or a mantra. This is the sixth limb of yoga, dharana (concentration).

RESTING AWARENESS. Settling awareness on one of the upper chakras— the heart, throat, third eye, or lower in the body at the womb. Here we have the opportunity to experience dhyana, or meditation.

SURRENDER. Allowing ourselves to dissolve into silence and spaciousness. Here we move from dhyana (possibly) toward samadhi, the final goal of yoga, and close to the fourth state (turiya). The latter can happen through grace. All of the previous steps help to prepare for this deepest level of surrender.

WELCOMING OURSELVES BACK. Moving back toward awareness of the gross plane. At this stage, we recognize where we are in space and time, deepen the breath, and remember that we have bodies. Our awareness begins to move from internal to external, hearing sounds, and moving the body as we welcome ourselves back to the "world."

SANKALPA SMIRTI. Remembering our sankalpa in the transition between the practice ending and waking.

FREEWRITING OR JOURNALING. Processing the experience through writing to deepen our understanding and cultivate memory and retentive power (*smirti*). This is when the practice of self-study can be most powerful; it is a way for us to record our insights and translate the wisdom from our practices.

GRATITUDE AND SELF-LOVE. Offering gratitude for the practice and love for yourself.

No matter their philosophies, all schools or lineages have one thing in common: *Nidra Shakti*. Uma Dinsmore-Tuli, one of the founders of the Yoga Nidra Network and the author of *Nidra Shakti: The Power of Rest—An Encyclopaedia of Yoga Nidra*, put it to me this way: "*Nidra Shakti* is a Sanskrit name that literally means 'the power of sleep.' This is the active ingredient of all yoga nidra, regardless of school or method. Nidra Shakti is the proper name of a form of the healing power of the deep feminine, as the goddess of sleep and rest who has the power to put everyone and everything, including the gods themselves, into a deep sleep."[27]

Let the teaching and practices become something for which you have great respect and love. Study, contemplate, and experiment. Let go of asking for permission to try to do it this way or that way and come to conclusions based on your own lived experience. At some point, the truth of the practice will begin to reveal itself to you. The key is to dedicate yourself to it for the clarity, wisdom, and stability it can provide. The practice is truly the teacher, and it will lead you to your true Self. Remember to be grateful.

· PART 2 ·

Welcoming Yoga Nidra

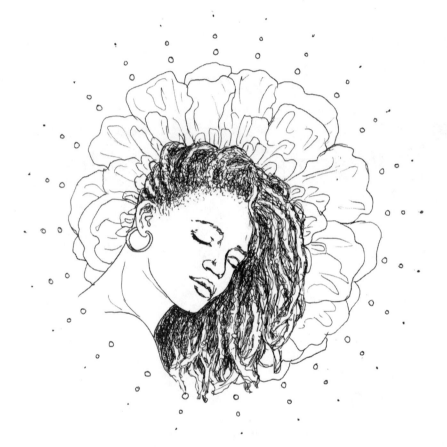

· 3 ·

What Does It Mean to Relax?

ONE OF THE FIRST THINGS I became aware of, as I began to practice and then share deep relaxation, was that it's difficult for most of us to "let go." Yoga teachers often give this instruction without the slightest consideration for how it will be received in a class full of people with varied life experiences and possible traumas. At the very least, life can be stressful, and over time it can create the type of tension that requires more than commanding ourselves to "let go" to relax.

It is hard to let go of the tension and constriction in the body and mind that have taken many years to accumulate. Some people say that "our issues live in our tissues," and Denise La Barre explains in her book, *Issues in Your Tissues,* what this means: "'Issues in your tissues' are emotions we haven't allowed ourselves to feel fully, or thoughts with a heavy emotional charge. As energetic residue in the body, they accumulate and build over time, starting first as tension and solidifying into disease according to our reactions to our life experiences."[1]

Deep relaxation practices help us to relax systematically and to bring awareness to all the parts of ourselves that require loving attention. Because we are taking a journey through the subtle body as we practice, that awareness may extend to our physical body, our thoughts, and even our beliefs. Unfortunately, it is a common tendency to identify with and hold on for dear life to parts of ourselves, like thoughts and beliefs, that lead to patterns of behavior that do not support our thriving. Remember the manomaya kosha. Because of our insecurities, fears, and biases, we may also hold on to ways of being that ensure that others cannot thrive, especially when we are in positions of power. This shows up as systemic racism, misogyny, or the mistreatment of others as a way to protect ourselves from perceived harm and scarcity.

Certain habits and thoughts may feel familiar and safe, and they can be reinforced by those around us, but that doesn't mean they aren't keeping us stuck. We may be scared that if we let go of these long-held ways of being, we will dissolve, even if they are causing us or others pain. The more we rely on what is familiar, the less we will grow. This recycling of suffering means that we have to learn the same lessons over and over again. This holding shows up everywhere in our lives, as tension in our bodies and our relationships and as an inability to move forward in life and in the collective as history repeating itself. If we can create an opportunity in our yoga nidra practice to create more awareness and ease within ourselves, it will be reflected outward in our lives.

HEALING TRAUMA WITH YOGA NIDRA

For many of us, the tension, stress, and emotional energy we're holding on to can be traced back to distressing or overwhelming events, known as psychological trauma. Trauma survivors who have practiced yoga nidra attest to its efficacy, with regular practice over time, at helping to loosen the hold that such events have on them. As mentioned in chapter 1, Richard Miller is largely to thank for the spread of yoga nidra practice outside of yoga studios. He's taken his iRest system into hospitals, military bases, prisons, and Head Start programs, to name a few, spurring interest in the research community to look for evidence to back up what anyone who has tried the practice already knows is true—that it works.

New studies continue to investigate yoga nidra's efficacy for those suffering from trauma, depression, and PTSD. A 2011 pilot study published in the *International Journal of Yoga Therapy* found that veterans with combat-related PTSD reported less rage, anxiety, and emotional reactivity and more feelings of relax ation, peace, self-awareness, and self-efficacy after eight weekly iRest sessions.[2] PTSD and trauma are complex topics of ongoing research. But early results support the theory and yogic teaching that consistent yoga nidra practice can help to improve the physical, mental, and emotional well-being of survivors.

If you are suffering from PTSD, depression, or trauma, it is important to investigate modalities and find teachers who not only understand and are educated in what you are experiencing, but who also promote agency and choice in your practice. The support of a therapist is invaluable when you are feeling overwhelmed, and many are now working on a sliding scale to make services more affordable for those in need. If you are a teacher of yoga nidra, it is important to educate yourself further about these conditions, address your own traumas, and begin with your own healing. You will find additional resources for this in the appendix.

NINE WAYS TO FIND MORE EASE IN YOUR PRACTICE

If you feel restless or struggle to settle in for deep relaxation or yoga nidra practices, there are things you can do to invite more ease into your practice when you feel difficult feelings arising. If you are a teacher, please consider experimenting with the following modifications so you can offer them to your students and community when needed.

1. Keep your eyes slightly open during practice.
2. Practice with a trusted person or pet in the room.
3. Physically touch or move the parts of your body that you would like to relax. Let go of the idea that you must "remain perfectly still."
4. Practice standing up. (Yes, you can.)
5. When practicing in a group, let the teacher know that you would like to find a spot in the room that feels safer for you instead of lining up or being contained in a circle formation.

6. Try a weighted blanket. It feels like a giant hug for the whole body. (Note: These blankets are said to ease anxiety, but they can also make some people feel confined, so test it out before making an investment.)

7. If complete silence makes you feel uneasy, experiment with adding sounds from nature, such as a rushing river or rain, soft wind chimes, crystal singing bowls, hang drums, or music you find soothing.

8. If lying on your back does not feel comfortable or sustainable over a long period of time, find a position that works for you, such as lying on your side or leaning against a wall facing the door with your eyes slightly open (see "Setting Up Your Nest" on page 87.

9. Remember that you have choices. Remember, you don't have to close your eyes if it feels uncomfortable. Leave the room if you need a break. You can also open your eyes with a soft focus and then return to the process. Work with a teacher on creating a safe place or inner resource. If something feels too uncomfortable, you can end the practice. Open your eyes and sit up as you mentally say to yourself, *I am choosing to end this practice now*. Try to take a few minutes to journal about your experience afterward.

IS IT SAFE?

Our bodies can hold on to the effects of stress for a long time, which can become a chronic low-level stress in itself. Stress can stem from anything—a demanding boss, a fight with a loved one, a struggle to secure childcare, a health scare, financial issues, politics, unmet basic needs, or trauma. For people living in Brown, Black, female, or LGBTQIA bodies, life may not feel safe, especially when there is a constant stream of evidence that safety is not always assured and in some cases intentionally denied. It doesn't feel safe to relax in a world that isn't welcoming to you, that labels you as lazy, that is oppressive, that can be a threat to your life in certain environments, and that is actually set up to make sure you don't thrive.

Research suggests that recent exposure to race-related stress can have a sustained impact on physiological stress responses for African Americans. Gail Parker, PhD, is a psychologist and yoga therapy educator and the author of *Restorative Yoga for Ethnic and Race-Based Stress and Trauma*. She reminded me that race-based stress and trauma are not the same as PTSD: "PTSD is regarded as a mental health disorder that is triggered by a life-threatening event that leaves the individual unable to shake off the trauma. Race-based stress is traumatic, but it is triggered by an external race-related event that causes emotional pain, not a threat to life, and unlike PTSD, it is recurrent, ongoing, and cumulative."

She added that this can all be further complicated by centuries-old intergenerational trauma, which is trauma inherited from our relatives. "It is important for people in Black and Brown bodies to know that feelings of relaxation or peacefulness can feel threatening to a nervous system that is conditioned to be on high alert. So learning to relax can seem stressful at first and takes time. The edge for people directly impacted by race-based stress and trauma isn't to push harder, it is to feel safe in stillness. To avoid retraumatizing others, we must each do our healing work as it relates to our own race and ethnicity."[3]

How far back can you trace your family tree? Some Native Americans believe that our actions affect the seven generations both before and after us. Our ancestral lineage makes us who we are. Even if we never met those long-ago relatives. Many times, we may experience a kind of psychic pain or restlessness that doesn't seem to belong to us. I have heard many students say they have felt a pain or sadness "that doesn't feel like mine." We are made up of so many stories from the past. We *all* have some form of trauma in our DNA. If that is true, we must also all carry the love, hope, and prayers of those who came before us. Many students have shared that they have felt the presence of loved ones or sensed that they were being "supported and protected" by their ancestors.

You may find it helpful to call your ancestors into a circle of healing. Extending your intentions for healing and rest to encompass your family lineage is a powerful way to explore forgiving, healing, and honoring those who came before you. We may have complicated relationships with our predecessors, from not knowing who they are or having been harmed by them to the knowledge that they were responsible for causing intentional suffering to large groups of people. For this reason, we can first begin by connecting to what the author of *Ancestral Medicine*, Daniel Foor, calls our "wise, kind and loving ancestors that are well in spirit."[4] This means connecting with those with whom you already feel relationship. If there aren't any humans that come to mind, you may want to include pets, spirit guides, or deities or connect to our collective and oldest ancestors: the earth, moon, sun, or stars.

Energy follows thought and prayers of healing, and love can reach as far and wide as we can imagine, beyond the confines of what we experience as linear time and space. Inviting ancestors into your practice for support and protection can help expand your experience of feeling supported and has the potential to extend healing deep into the roots of your family tree.

OCTAVIA'S STORY

Octavia Raheem is a yoga teacher and the author of the book *Gather*. She finds the practice of inviting her ancestors to rest along with her in yoga nidra practice to be a powerful experience.

When I first began to practice stillness-based yoga (restorative, yoga nidra, meditation), I encountered a kind of restlessness that was shocking. I encountered resistance to pausing. I even met a sense of fear that "something" bad would happen if I allowed myself to lay down. It was as if I worried about being "caught" resting.

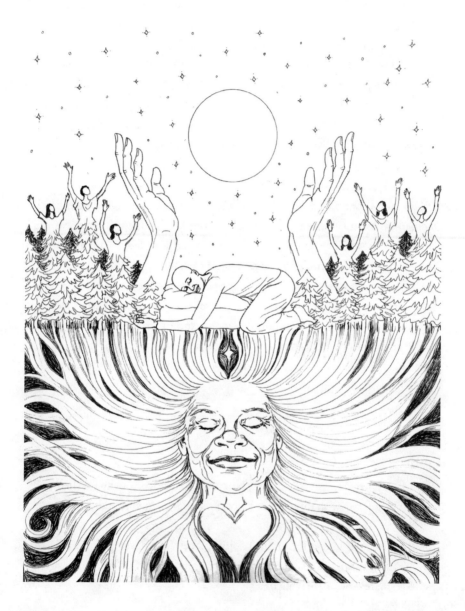

I reflected on my conditioning: *Girl . . . you better work twice as hard, be twice as fast, stay twice as long, and maybe, JUST maybe, you will have half of a chance as others.* That conditioning came from my mother and her mother and her mother and is rooted in very real experiences.

That restlessness brought me into direct awareness that I didn't know how to rest and had never seen anyone in my family rest. I'd lay down in those early restorative yoga classes and toss and turn. I may have even broken a sweat from the discomfort of "doing nothing." In a visceral way I knew my restlessness was a symptom of being severely tired, not only from my life but from the lives of the women who gave me life. Stillness awakened me to how much generational weariness and bone-deep ancestral fatigue I carried.

It sounds poetic, yet history, family, and cultural stories tell us that Black women in America have been treated, as Zora Neale Hurston wrote, as the "mule of the world." Ridden, worked, and forced into labor—birthing, domestic, field, and beyond until we ran out of fuel, breath, or life.

When I practice restorative yoga, yoga nidra, or meditation and "go inside," I meet the most fatigued parts of myself and invite those parts to rest. I know how to work. Rest requires devotion and practice on my part. I also call in an ancestor who I know toiled through her whole life and could never acknowledge she was tired. I rest in honor of the women within me who were denied the opportunity to rest.[5]

· Ancestral Circle of Healing ·

[5 minutes]

If you feel called to honor your ancestors in your practice, you can honor them and request protection with this exercise before you begin your yoga nidra practice.

1. Lie down in a comfortable position. Feel your navel rise and fall as you inhale and exhale. Feel your body resting on the floor or whatever you are lying on.

2. Scan the body from the tips of your toes to the top of your head, noticing which parts are touching the floor. Feel the points of contact.
3. Scan the body again for those parts that are not touching the floor.
4. Feel the body as a whole of all its parts.
5. Draw a circle of protective light around the body.
6. Call around you the guides or ancestors with whom you feel relationship and that are supportive energies. Invite only energies that are benevolent and loving. Ask them to establish a layer of support and protection around the outer circumference of your circle of light.
7. Feel that your ancestors are helping to cleanse the space around you. Feel and know that you are protected.

Take a moment to dedicate your practice to all your ancestors and to their healing. Thank them for persevering in their lives, the very lives that allowed you to be born. Feel gratitude for the miracle of life, the breath. Notice it, one breath at a time. Remember that it is your birthright to breathe, to rest, and to rise in power. Feel the support of the earth, your guides, and your ancestors. Be present to the breath for 3 minutes, feel the belly rise and fall, and let yourself be held. Know that you are being blessed, guided, supported, and protected.

SELF-INQUIRY

1. What relationship do you have with your ancestors or family lineage?
2. What is your understanding of how trauma might be present in your lineage?
3. Take a few minutes, or as long as you need, to freewrite about any emotions or feelings that arise when you consider the lives of those who came before you.

4. How can you honor the lives of your ancestors and those who will be future ancestors?

A REST IN PROGRESS

Many of us have narratives in our DNA that tell us it is not safe to relax and let go. The science of epigenetics has begun to show in recent years how various factors in our lives and lifestyles—such as diet, exercise, and even trauma—can modify DNA by switching genes on or off. A 2018 study found that the sons of Union army soldiers who'd endured severe hardship as prisoners of war (POWs) during the Civil War were more likely to die young than were the POWs' daughters or the sons of veterans who hadn't been POWs. With controls for other factors that might have influenced the sons' longevity, this study suggests that the fathers' trauma left a mark on their genes that was then passed down to their sons.[6]

Feeling a lack of safety also can be tied to our ancestral background. Exploring our family history—which might include war, slavery, genocide, the Holocaust, domestic abuse, and events that we have absolutely no way of knowing about—can give us new understanding and compassion for ourselves and others. The key is to empower ourselves by finding the best way to honor all the parts of us that show up for the practice with self-love. Self-love helps us to move beyond the limits that others have placed on us.

Sonja, a yoga nidra teacher in Australia, says the practice helped her to open a doorway to new possibilities, but she still struggles to surrender fully. Born into a working-class Scottish family in the 1970s, her home life was chaotic and difficult:

My maternal ancestors were all domestic servants across the ages in Scotland and Ireland—a tough existence in often harsh climates. I was always intellectually curious, but I was often reminded where I was from . . . and told "not to get above my station." I struggle to surrender, to rest, to find ease, as everything was always hard [for them]. Very little came with ease. I was raised to work hard. I was not raised to pause and take a rest. Learning to ask for what I need is a continual work in progress.

As Sonja is learning though her yoga nidra practice, she deserves to rest and to experience the grace of yoga nidra, but there is still resistance. It is important for us to be aware of our resistance and to notice how it shows up in practice and in our lives.

SELF-INQUIRY

Please take some time to consider the following questions and how they may inform your practices.

1. Who, if anyone, modeled how to rest and practice self-care and self-love for you?
2. What message did you receive about the worth of rest and your ability to have it as an integral part of your life?
3. What habits, thoughts, or resistance prevent you from fully "dropping in" to the practice?
4. If part of your legacy were to change the relationship to rest and self-care for your family lineage, how would you begin?

THE RELAXATION RESPONSE

You've probably heard of the fight-or-flight mode, in which the body senses danger and releases hormones and chemicals to increase heart rate, breathing rate, blood pressure, metabolic rate, and blood flow to the muscles, prepping the body to either defend itself or escape. This physiological reaction to stress was essential for evolutionary survival, but in modern life, it can be triggered by something as mundane as an full inbox. Those of us who are affected by PTSD or trauma can spend a lot of time in this state, with elevated blood pressure and heart rate, ready to go to battle. It can be difficult to shut it off.

In 1975 Herbert Benson, MD, now a director emeritus of mind/body medicine at Harvard, released the groundbreaking book *The Relaxation Response*. By studying meditators, Benson discovered that humans are essentially able to flip a switch and move out of fight-or-flight mode supported by the sympathetic nervous system and into rest-and-digest mode, activating the parasympathetic nervous system. He called it the "relaxation response."[7] Decades before #selfcaresaturday, Benson was talking about self-care and finally backing up with science something that yogis have known for thousands of years.

When we spend time in the rest-and-digest state, the body heals, rejuvenates, and digests on both a mental and physical level. You might notice that once you lie down and get comfortable in Savasana, your stomach starts to growl. This is a clear sign that the body is moving toward a place of rest-and-digest.

Through his research, Benson identified a few things that needed to be present to activate the relaxation response:

- A quiet environment
- A prayer repeated silently or aloud
- A comfortable position
- A passive attitude of "not worrying about how well one is performing the technique and simply putting aside distracting thoughts to return to one's focus."[8]

Most of Benson's requirements are present when we do the practice of yoga nidra. This tells us that our practice offers us the tools to begin exploring how we can affect our autononic nervous system, the part of the nervous system responsible for control of bodily functions that are not consciously directed like the heartbeat and breathing.

In yoga nidra, we use body sensing and breath awareness as first steps to the practice. It's no wonder that we quite often get so relaxed that we fall asleep when we do deep relaxation practices. It is possible to feel less anxious and stressed after just 10 to 15 minutes of deep relaxation, especially when we bring focus to our breathing and begin to move our awareness inward as the first steps toward relaxation. Our parasympathetic nervous system is activated, and the body senses that it can begin to let go.

Yoga nidra—along with other quiet practices like yin yoga, restorative yoga, gentle yoga, and sound baths—is one of the fastest-growing practices in yoga studios today. This indicates that the world at large knows it needs rest and a connection to the quiet dynamism that lives within. For those of us who feel called to share passive practices, it is of the utmost importance that we are rested and have spent extensive time dedicated to practicing. It doesn't matter if you are sharing practices in your living room with family and friends or in front of a hundred people. The transmission of a powerful experience of deep relaxation begins when a teacher embodies the moonlike vibrations of nurturing, peace, calm, and stillness.

As the person receiving the practice, all that's being asked of you is to let go of "doing" and be guided by grace back to the Source of who you really are, your true Self. The multilineage yoga nidra educator and founder of Tri-Being, John Vosler, offered this reflection:

> It's a non-doing practice, a practice of subtraction, you don't have to do anything or make anything happen. You can't make an experience happen, you ARE the experience, you are the vibration of the source.[9]

SELF-INQUIRY

Please take a moment to consider that some specific things or environments make you feel most relaxed. Take some time to answer the following questions to contemplate your relationship with relaxation.

1. Describe what it feels like in your body when you are experiencing relaxation.
2. Name three things that need to be present in your environment to invoke a peaceful feeling.
3. Do you have a prayer or mantra that brings you peace?
4. Is there a special place that you have visited that evokes a sense of peace within you? Describe it in detail, write a poem about it, or draw it, remembering all the relaxing and peaceful elements of this place.

The following exercise will help you explore and experience where tension may be present in your body. It will also help you to learn where the physical body may need extra support when setting yourself up for longer practices. It is a simple but powerful practice that helps to illuminate where resistance is present in the body.

· Body Awareness Exercise ·
[5 minutes]

Notice how you feel when you begin and notice how you feel afterward. Do this practice for a few consecutive days to develop more awareness and understanding of your body.

1. Lie down in Savasana (Corpse Pose, page 183. Notice your breathing. Feel your navel rising on the inhalation and falling on the exhalation. (2 minutes)
2. Begin to move your attention slowly through your body as you follow your gentle breath. Scan from your toes to the top of your head, and take a few breaths at each body part, starting at your feet. (3 minutes)

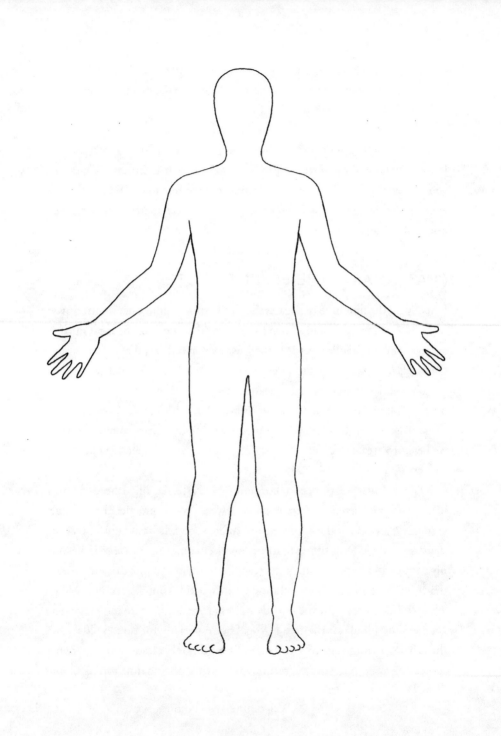

3. Notice where you feel constriction in your body. Breathe into those constricted areas. Soften and relax. Make mental notes of where you feel tension. (1 minute)

Make notes on the body outline shown on page 65 or draw your own in your journal. Where did you feel tension, constriction, or tightness? Where did you feel pain? Where did you feel the most flow or freedom? Did you feel any emotion or thoughts arise as you visited certain body parts? What did you notice about your breath?

PRATYAHARA: THE ESSENTIAL STEP

Pratyahara, the fifth limb of yoga, is the ability to withdraw our attention away from the outside world and into our inner world. It is one of the most important elements of practice, yet it is the least explored. Pratyahara is the bridge that leads us to touching our inner radiance. We receive information through the gates of the five senses: sight, hearing, touch, smell, and taste. Those senses usually pull our attention outside ourselves. But with practice, we can draw those senses inward. When we can practice using the senses to move inward, we begin to create a foundation for deeper practice and open new portals of awareness.

When I first began deep relaxation practices, I felt like I needed a perfectly quiet and serene environment to have a "good" practice. I would get annoyed if anyone in the house made a single sound. It wasn't until I realized that I should let go of trying to direct outer circumstances that were beyond my control and instead manage my reaction to them and move deeper inward that I was able to practice in a house with two kids running around. After a while, I didn't even hear the outside noises anymore. Developing pratyahara is an essential limb on the tree of yoga, but especially for householders and those living in noisy environments. This is the limb that leads us to experience something as deep as yoga nidra, and it's worth spending time tuning up our relationship with pratyahara. Try the following practice to awaken your power of pratyahara.

Using the information you learned in the Body Awareness Exercise, consider what props, such as a blanket, a pillow, or bolsters, you may want to have handy. Refer back to your notes and experiment with how best to support your body. If your physical body is uncomfortable, it will be difficult to draw your awareness inward.

· Pratyahara Practice ·

[10–15 minutes]

1. Lie down in Savasana (Corpse Pose, page 183) or sit in a chair with your eyes open. Feel the breath move into and out of your body through your nostrils. Feel the skin inside your nose being caressed by the breath, noticing the temperature of the in-breath and the out-breath and the difference between them. (2 minutes)
2. Move into two-pronged awareness: watch yourself breathe while also being aware that there is another part of you that is watching from a different perspective, as though you are watching yourself in a movie.
3. Continue being aware of the breath, now watching your navel rise on inhalations and fall on exhalations. (2 minutes) Keep your eyes open, notice what you see in your physical surroundings.
4. Close your eyes and notice the darkness (3 seconds), then gently open your eyes about halfway and notice the light filtering through. (3 seconds)
5. As you open and close your eyes, notice what you feel or sense in your body. Now close your eyes and look into the darkness beyond your eyelids. Place an eye pillow over your eyes (if it feels safe and comfortable to do so). Let your awareness rest in the darkness. (2 minutes)

6. Keeping your eyes closed, continue to notice the rise and fall of your belly. Continue to be aware that you are breathing while simultaneously being aware that there is a part of you that is watching you, watch yourself breathe. Become aware of awareness. (2 minutes)

7. Let your attention travel to sound. Listen for the farthest sounds you can possibly hear. (30 seconds)

8. Continue being aware of awareness. (30 seconds)

9. Let your attention jump from sound to sound to sound, letting go of identifying what the sounds are and just letting your attention move. Begin to draw your awareness of sound closer and closer to you. Hear the sound of your breath, then the sound of your heart beating and the blood and fluids moving through your body. Now just let go of the awareness of sounds. Let all sounds be out there in the distance. Feel as though you are in the center of a circle, and all the sounds are outside the circle. (2 minutes)

10. Feel your body lying on the ground (or on your chair). Notice all the body parts that are touching the floor (or chair). As you scan your body for these points of contact, go slowly and actually feel each point. Feel your body being magnetized toward the earth through these points. (2 minutes)

11. Now feel the space between your body and the floor. Feel the space around your body. Feel yourself as the space around your body. Rest in awareness. (2 minutes)

12. Remember that part of you was there before you had a body. (1 minute)

13. Remember that part of you was there when the world was created. (1 minute)

14. Rest in the knowing that you are eternal. (1 minute)

15. Slowly coming back, notice the sounds around you.

16. Bring awareness back to the body and deepen your breath, remaining still.
17. Notice your body breathing, remember where you are—the room, building. Welcome yourself back.
18. Begin to open your eyes and complete the practice with 3 minutes of freewriting.

Moving into a space where you withdraw your awareness may make you feel vulnerable, and you may be called to add an energetic layer of protection around your body. The following practice can help.

· Energetic Protection Practice ·
[5 minutes]

This practice may feel supportive in certain environments such as group classes or unfamiliar practice spaces to establish a level of energetic protection around you.

1. Once you are in your desired position to practice yoga nidra, close your eyes and visualize that you are drawing a circle of protective energy around your body. You can create this circle out of any substance that you feel nurtures you—water, moonlight, the energy of love.[10] Feel as though this circle emanates healing power toward you; you may feel cocooned by its presence, bathed in the vibration of healing. (1 minute)
2. Next, draw another circle around that circle. Visualize that this second circle protects you from any unwanted energy from others. Create that unbroken circle using anything you choose, such as fire or white light. (1 minute)
3. Now visualize the third circle of protective energy around you. This one protects you from any thoughts that might disturb your

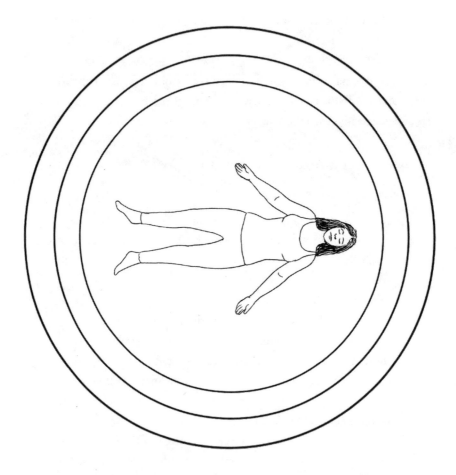

practice; for now, you can leave them outside the rings. As hard as they may try, they cannot get in. See them being neutralized, put to sleep by the ring of energy around you. (1 minute)

4. Feel a sense of peace and protection as you visualize, feel, or sense yourself inside the center of these three circles.[11] (2 minutes)

SELF-INQUIRY

Remember that your history, lineage, and social location have so much to do with the messages that have infiltrated your beliefs about what you are capable of and what you deserve. They also factor greatly in your actual ability to access the resources that can help you to step into your birthright of abundance, empowerment, and true freedom. None of this is your fault. You can start by envisioning something different for yourself.

In fact, it might be scary to think about what life would look like if you were living in a way that honored your potential. The teaching of tantra tells us that if we want to see shifts in the outer world, we can begin with the universe inside us. When we begin to change our own energy and thoughts, that can have an influence on how life can show up for us. This isn't about magical thinking; it's about getting clear on your goals and envisioning how to reclaim your birthright to thrive.

1. What are three things in your life that would change if you were well rested?

2. What have you learned about the value of rest in the last twelve months?

3. What are three things that bring you joy for which you would like to cultivate more time and energy in your life?

4. Do you feel that you deserve to relax deeply? Why or why not? Explain in detail.

5. If you said that you didn't deserve rest, can you remember an

experience or time in your life when you learned that resting or relaxing had a negative effect?

6. How can you support yourself or engage others to help support you so you can take on relaxation as a consistent practice? Is there anything that you waste time doing that you can replace with yoga nidra practice?

RELAXATION VOW

If you feel ready to commit to honoring your birthright to rest, relax, and awaken spiritually, you can make a vow to yourself to rest. The following is a suggestion of how to structure one; adapt it and make it your own. You can write the vow in your journal, create an art piece inspired by it, frame it, and place it on your altar.

I remember that deep relaxation, rest, and freedom are my birthright. I commit to the practices that lead me to know the deepest parts of myself. I effortlessly remain awake and aware during the transitions in life. I recognize every transition as a sacred portal that leads to my truth, power, and wisdom.

I commit to this practice because I _____
_____.

My wish for myself through this practice is _____
_____
_____.

I commit to practicing deep relaxation and yoga nidra _____
times per week.

Signed _____

· 4 ·

The Householder's Flow

Householder's Prayer

The altar is in my heart.
The sun and the moon are my gurus.
I trust the earth to support me.
Each time I close my eyes, I enter the void.
My heart is the portal to my sacred cave.
I whisper the names of the Divine as I prepare my meals.
I notice the flow of my beloveds' breath as they fall asleep,
and I synchronize my breath to the flow of love.
I place a blessing in the pause between the breaths.
I hold the power to create a new reality with every thought.
I honor silence as a blessing.
I explore who I am and who I am not in the mirror of relationship.
I question my beliefs with curiosity and courage.
I honor my ancestors.
I lay down all self-doubt with compassion and forgiveness.
I remember the light of my soul as I enter the dream state.
I recall the beauty of truth as I transition from sleep to waking.
I know the vibration of truth.
I remember that nothing is mundane.
I honor the power of the transition as a portal to transformation
Everything is an offering. My life is a sacred ritual.

—Tracee Stanley

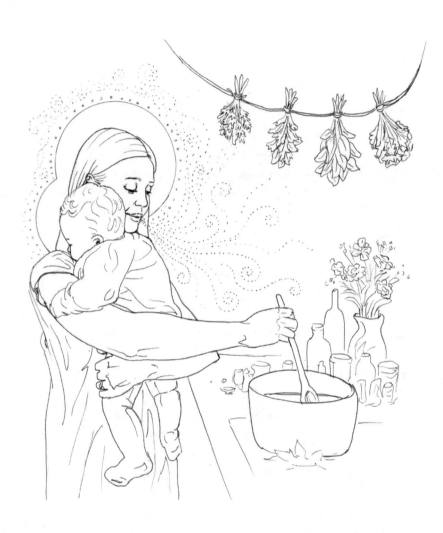

DURING MY MORE THAN twenty years of teaching, the obstacle that people have consistently shared as standing in the way of their practice is time. When I first began practicing yoga over twenty-five years ago, I had plenty of time to practice. Back then, the workday ended the moment you left the office, most people didn't have cell phones, and no one dared to call you at dinnertime because they knew it was family time.

For most of us today, that scenario seems like a dream. In fact, just trying to get people to put their phones down during a meal can seem like a chore. According to a recent survey, 71 percent of us are sleeping with our phones— in our hands, in our beds, or at least within reach on our nightstands.[1] We have created lives where our attention focuses on the external, gathering data and information, seeking validation through "likes," and succumbing to intense FOMO (fear of missing out) that makes it hard to turn off the devices that link us to the outside world 24/7. This existence leaves very little room for exploration of our internal landscape, devotion to practice, spiritual study, the things that bring us joy or relaxation just for the sake of our own sanity and well-being.

MAKING CHOICES

Tech companies are banking on the fact that we would rather distract ourselves than be present to life. This was evident during "stay-at-home" orders at the beginning of the 2020 COVID-19 pandemic, when people ran to platforms like Instagram, Zoom, and Netflix to the point that they became overloaded and kept crashing. We are constantly making choices. But what influences the choices we make moment to moment? This reminds me of the simple but profound concept of desire and the idea that the seed of every thought, deed, and action is desire.

The Indian spiritual teacher, author, and scholar Eknath Easwaran translated this powerful verse from the Brihadaranyaka Upanishad: "You are what your deep, driving desire is. As your desire is, so is your will. As your will is, so is your deed. As your deed is, so is your destiny."[2] When we consistently make choices that deny the importance of our inner lives in exchange for the things that are continually changing and not a real source of truth, we keep looking outward for validation and meaning. It's called distraction, and by succumbing to it, we are giving our power away. All the energy that we possess is being dispersed and wasted in chasing things that can never bring us lasting happiness.

If we can begin to explore the source of our desires, we will realize that they have the power to radically shape our lives. Next time you notice that you are procrastinating or allowing yourself to be distracted with things that waste time, ask yourself, *What am I avoiding? What am I denying myself by not being present? How do my actions contribute to my feelings of being overwhelmed by my life? How is this behavior shaping my life? Am I willing to change?* In a life that may include any combination of partners, jobs, kids, homework, family, pets, bills, aging parents, or building a business, we have so much to take care of just to get by. But the distractions keep coming— impulse shopping, internet scrolling, social media, online dating, or overindulging in general. The question is, what is it we are being distracted from? The answer is easy: our power.

No matter how shiny those distractions are, they are not more brilliant than the eternal light that makes its home within you. Perhaps you have intuitively sensed that there is something more to who you are beyond what you see, that there is a part of you that is vibrant and thriving. Maybe you feel like you've lost that part of yourself under all of life's overwhelming demands. But yogic wisdom tells us that the thriving, vibrant radiance is who we are, and it is eternal; it's a light that never goes out. Remember the light inside the innermost tiny nesting doll? That light is your power source, your own unique ray of brilliance.

Nischala Joy Devi translated my favorite Patanjali's sutra 1.36, *viśokā va jyotiṣmatī*, as saying, "Cultivate devotion to the supreme, ever-blissful light within."[3] This sutra refers to a light within us that is beyond all sorrow, that is unaffected by our conditioning or life experiences. It is not tainted in any way. It is pure, blissful, and eternal. It was there before you had a name and will be there when you no longer have a body. I believe that part of our purpose in life is to taste this radiance. The remembrance of this radiance is one of the gifts of yoga nidra. In many yoga traditions, a light is said to reside inside the "cave," or deepest recesses, of the heart. Remember that one of the sacred portals is the heart center.

Unfortunately, we give ourselves no chance of experiencing this inner light (think, the innermost nesting doll) when our focus is constantly directed outward. It might feel like modern life leaves us no choice but to be externally focused—unless we're living in a cave somewhere. When we are living the life of a householder, which I define as those of us with duties and obligations to our families, jobs, parents, or pets, it can feel like there is little to no time for practice. You might fantasize about going to meditate in a cave and leaving all of your responsibilities behind. But what if instead your life as a householder held keys to your evolution? It can.

It was vital for me to present this book in a way that incorporates practice for the householders—especially since most of us are not living in caves. The chapters in this part are meant to inspire you to reframe what your devoted practice looks like and to give you tools to carry on a practice no matter what life events present themselves.

REDEFINING PRACTICE

I wrote the poem at the beginning of this chapter to remind myself that I have space and I have time, no matter how fast life is moving and how many things there are to do. I can always find moments during the day that connect me to my practice if I elevate my view of everyday life as not separate from my spiritual practice. If the poem resonates with you, you might consider printing it out and placing it on your altar (you'll learn how to create one in chapter 5) as a reminder that you already have everything you need to practice. Because you do. Many times we look at spiritual teachers or "gurus" and think they are living "high up on the mountain," untouched by the world. This is problematic because the world will change while they are up there in the clouds, and we may then be left with teachers who are out of touch or seemingly uncaring about the problems faced by those of us living a spiritual yet very worldly life. Having discernment about the teachers we choose and cultivating a relationship with our inner wisdom has never been more important.

If we can reframe how we see practice and use the myriad opportunities that daily life gives us to do that practice, we won't need to long for a cave or an ashram. Life becomes our practice, and we can take refuge at the altars of our hearts. Our practice reminds us that life is sacred, and we can experience the quality of radiance in our daily lives.

I recently saw a man in a workshop in Vancouver scowling at me when I asked the group to join me in committing to a forty-day practice. I felt his frustration and said, "Are you wondering how the heck you're going to fit this into your life?" He replied, "Yeah. I have five kids, and I'm a stay-at-home dad. There's no way I'm going to be able to practice every day. It was a stretch for me just to be here for one day." I felt a deep well of emotion rising within him. He desperately wanted to have time to dedicate to a consistent practice, and he was frustrated and sad that he couldn't see a way to do that.

I suggested to him and the group that we reframe the idea of what yoga practice looks like—more specifically, who a dedicated yoga practitioner is. Usually when we think of dedicated yoga practitioners, we visualize people who have many hours a day to meditate, study, and practice. We see them as very disciplined. They always seem to be reading the scriptures, discovering new teachers, trying new modalities, and going to workshops or on spiritual pilgrimages. This kind of time is a luxury and a privilege and not the case for most of us. We consider ourselves lucky if we can eke out time for a class once or twice a week. Somehow, we have gotten the idea that spiritual fruits are only delivered to those who have a lot of time, resources, and discipline to dedicate to practice. We decide that if we can't do a full hour of practice, it's not worth even bothering. But who said that a "practice" needed to be an hour or 90 minutes to be valid? That comes from the commercialization of yoga as a wellness product to be sold and not as a lifelong practice that can lead to spiritual freedom.

It's true that it can be a little daunting when you read in texts, such as the Yoga Sutras, that say the way to practice yoga is with consistency, for a long period of time, with no interruption.

With no interruption? For most of us, that is a nonstarter. We feel like we are set up to fail; it's easy to give up or not even begin. Let's drop the idea that a practice needs to be an hour just because that is what yoga studios have been selling us for years. What if we stopped compartmentalizing and saw the whole of our lives as a spiritual practice? What if we explored the many opportunities during the day that can connect us to a deeper part of ourselves? What if that became our practice?

Try seeing your practice as a twenty-four-hour cycle. Each breath, mantra, pose, mudra, or contemplation you are able to thread into your day makes up your Householder's Flow. Your twenty-four-hour practice can flow through all the states of consciousness: waking, dreaming, and deep sleep. Let it become the fabric that supports you as you take care of family, commute to work, prepare for a meeting, do classes online, bathe your children, and prepare for a night's sleep.

If you really want to have a dedicated practice, it's as simple as making the choice, then figuring out how that choice can fit your life. Let go of any comparison to what you think "practice" should be like and tune in to how you want it to feel. Be honest about what is possible for you.

The Yoga Sutras tells us that we should practice with steadiness and ease. Most of the time, we think of this as steadiness in our physical posture and letting go of effort as a form of surrender. But what happens when we are not practicing asana? Is it possible to adapt steadiness and ease into our daily lives? Learning how to bring a sense of steadiness into the ever-changing ebb and flow that occurs during each day and finding small ways to keep the sacred thread of our practice running through everything we do is the key to the Householder's Flow. You can connect to steadiness by remembering the part of you that is eternal. Remember what it is that you have unwavering faith in. If you feel like you don't have faith right now, consider what you would like to have faith in. Contemplate what it means to be awake to this sacred thread in every moment. Let discipline transform into devotion and your life will be a sacred ritual.

The practice of yoga nidra attunes us to the transitions between the waking, dreaming, and deep sleep states. The transitions are where the power and the magic lie; each one is a little space of the void. There are many transitions throughout the day. If we can begin to be aware of these transitions, we can use them to stay more awake and present to our practice and to the little nidra moments every day.

As householders, we can turn every sunrise, every breath, every pause between the breath into a sacred portal into practice. The most potent portals are the moments when you are about to fall asleep and awaken. Just by using the simple 3- to 5-minute practices I've included in the practice chapters as a start and end to your day, you will create a twenty-four-hour flow of practice that can begin to give your waking life a new color—one of presence and grace. You may find your relationship to time and practice beginning to shift, and my hope is that you will then be able to incorporate the longer deep relaxation practices too.

PARENTHOOD AND PRACTICE

I met a woman at a retreat in Austin who had completed a very rigorous yoga therapist training program and was getting back to her practice after five years away. She felt that when her child was born, she began to "lose the cushion between experiencing something and reacting to it." Her years of practice had given her the ability to slow down and notice how she reacted to things and to be more present overall. She was able to delay reacting and to respond with better choices. But all the hours of practice and study hadn't prepared her for motherhood and maintaining a consistent practice while caring for her child. Little by little, she "watched that cushion of sanity getting smaller and smaller until one day it was gone." She felt she had lost her practice and her clarity.

This is a feeling we can probably all relate to, as at one time or another, something we were doing consistently that made us feel great and healthy somehow got derailed and then eventually disappeared from our lives. Months later, we find ourselves thinking that we have to get back to it and we don't know how. Another habit or responsibility has taken its place. I would say that this woman hadn't really "lost" her practice. It was waiting for her in abeyance, like a forgotten bank account waiting for her to claim the funds. Her practice needed a radical reframing.

What kind of practice can you do when the baby finally falls asleep, and you have so many other essential things to do like take a shower or prepare a meal for yourself? The answer is whatever you can. The practice chapters include short mini practices that can be done in 3 to 5 minutes. They are all portals into deeper states of awareness and sacred living while taking care of day-to-day demands.

Ashley, a new mother of a one-year-old, told me, "Once you don't have as much time, everything that is unimportant falls away. You become clear that everything is a choice. You become more discerning." In this way, the perception of lack of time can be one of the gems of parenthood. It allows us to practice detachment, to examine the root of our desires, and to sharpen our discernment. We can use the feeling of "no time" to get clear on what we want our lives to be about. We get to create new paradigms around how, where, and when we practice; to rediscover what a personal devoted practice looks and *feels* like for us; and to explore what our practice means for those around us. Kate Northrup, the author of *Do Less*, a mother of two, and a successful entrepreneur, says yoga nidra helped her with mental clarity and physical energy: "I felt like I had gone into a state of deeper stillness and calm than I had experienced in a long time."[4]

We get to reclaim that calm as a householder when we reinvent for ourselves what practice looks like. I have a dear friend, Bill, who has been practicing meditation in his car for over fifteen years. Every morning he goes into his garage, sits in his parked car, and does his meditation practice. His car is where he finds peace. It is comfortable, quiet, and free of distraction. He has turned his car into a meditation cave.

It's important here to give yourself permission to find creative ways to see what works for you and what doesn't. The more open you are to experimenting with little increments of time during the day, the more your practice will strengthen and blossom. Here are some tips to get you started. Choose one that resonates and start with that as a way to find your unique flow. Over time you can add others until you find what works best for your situation.

FIFTEEN STEPS TO GET INTO THE TWENTY-FOUR-HOUR HOUSEHOLDER'S FLOW

1. Let go of the idea that your practice needs to be 15, 30, or 90 minutes long to be meaningful or valid.

2. Instead of one long practice, try 2- to 3-minute mini practice portals that you can weave throughout your day. You can set the timer on your phone to remind you when to practice. Find time to lay down and practice the Body Awareness Exercise on page 64 or Pratyahara Practice on page 67 for 3 minutes. When you do have a few minutes of space to practice, notice how resistance to resting or practicing may show up. Be aware of what you feel called to do instead. Is it nurturing, supportive, or healing? Is your default mode moving you toward healing or toward distraction and staying stuck?

3. Use your least favorite chore as a portal to practice. Chant, sing, or follow your breath while washing dishes, doing your taxes, doing laundry, or mopping the floor. Use your resistance as a way

to turn the mundane into the sacred. You will find suggestions for mantras in the resources, but any song or affirmation that is offered with devotion will work.

4. Leave a small space in your home—a chair, your yoga mat, a corner of a room, a closet, or even your car—set up and ready for your practice. Begin to see every seat as a potential meditation seat or yoga nidra nest. (You'll learn how to set yourself up for the ultimate surrender in the next chapter.)

5. Acknowledge your obstacles. Let go of being surprised and frustrated when they show up. Observe the barriers to practice that arise and the obstacles that you place in your own way. Be aware of which patterns keep showing up. How can you shift something to create a new outcome?

6. Remember that all the practices you do, no matter how small they may seem, are preparing you for deep relaxation, yoga nidra, and *truth*.

7. Decide what you are willing to commit to.

8. Connect to the desire in your heart to deepen your practice and let that be what guides you. Even when you feel like you cannot "do" a single thing, connecting to that longing with a sense of gratitude that the fire is burning within you will support you. Connect to it with gratitude, as opposed to despair and disappointment that the desire has not yet been fulfilled; know that you are moving toward it. Connect with your faith that things can change. Remember the cycles of nature where nothing is permanent. There is a season for everything.

9. Be creative. Look for the pauses, transitions, spaciousness, and silence. The day is full of natural transitions: sunrise, high noon, sunset, moonrise. Use these natural transitions to remind you to pause. When you pause, you create a natural void, so place a mantra, an affirmation, a bible verse, or a blessing for yourself in that

space to empower yourself. These are the little nidra moments that will change your relationship to the practice.

10. Use every relationship as a mirror to understand more about yourself. Notice your reactions and what beliefs you hold on to. Be willing to see another point of view as a way toward understanding. Examine conflicts and ask yourself, *Could I have created a more healing outcome for all involved? What am I not willing to admit about myself? What systems or conditions are present that prevent me from thriving and what resources are available to me for assistance?*

11. Find at least one friend who is like-minded with whom you can connect to share insights and experiences. Even if it's a text to say, "I had a tough day today," or "I meditated in my closet today," or "I removed some apps from my phone so I would have more time to practice—I can't believe I didn't do it sooner." Use technology as a way to support your practice instead of as a distraction.

12. Reframe your deep relaxations and yoga nidra practices as surrenders. Remind yourself, *It's time to surrender* instead of *It's time to practice.* Let go of the energy of doing. Yoga nidra is a practice of non-doing, and grace descends when you let go.

13. Set up an altar at home. (Keep reading to learn more about how.) Let it be a reminder to pause at least once a day and remember your commitment to yourself.

14. When you notice negative thoughts, replace them with kindness and compassion. Study and practice Yoga Sutra 2:33, translated by Pandit Rajmani Tigunait as "to arrest conflicting thoughts, cultivate thoughts opposed to them."[5] This is said to be a way toward a peaceful mind. It also helps us become aware of our thoughts.

15. As soon as you wake up, bring awareness to the flow of your breath for 1 minute. Even if you have a child who wakes you up, you have a moment to say to yourself, *What is my breathing like? Let me bring awareness to my breathing, feeling my navel rise and fall, while I am also bringing attention to my child. Can I hold the feeling of inner peace while experiencing that a part of my attention is also being directed externally?* Parents are the best multitaskers around. You can do this!

16. Be aware of the phases of the moon, taking just one moment each night to see the moon in the night sky. Remembering the phase from the night before, see if you can imagine the current moon phase in your mind's eye prior to looking up. Offer a prayer, a blessing, or gratitude for her cooling light. Notice how you feel at each moon phase; look for patterns and take notes. Learn the last verse of Ratri Suktum (p. 188).

SELF-INQUIRY

1. Recall a time when you directed all of your will to one thing. What was it? How did it feel? How did it change you? How can you tap into that force of will within you to commit to reframing your practice to a twenty-four-hour Householder's Flow?

2. What do you have faith in? How can this help to shape and support your practice?

3. Is there someone in your household you can ask for support so you can take 3 minutes a few times during the day to do mini practices?

4. How are you careless or forgetful? When do you "check out"? Can you bring more presence and purpose into your daily activities?

· 5 ·

How to Prepare for Yoga Nidra

WHAT DO YOU THINK of when you hear the word *nest*? Better yet, what do you feel in your body? I think of feeling cocooned, warm, cozy, nurtured, held, and healed. The yoga nidra nest is a gift to yourself. Remember, you deserve it.

Uma Dinsmore-Tuli introduced me to the concept of the yoga nidra nest. She encouraged us in a workshop to fully embrace the feminine (the qualities of nurturing, relaxation, and support) and to make ourselves divinely comfortable with cozy blankets, props, and adequate support to allow our bodies to release and let go into the earth beneath us. This kind of setup was a far cry from lying on a hard floor with a simple yoga mat and a serape that barely covered my feet or shoulders. That's how I had been practicing for years. And there were always parts of my body that would begin to feel very heavy, cold, uncomfortable, and sometimes painful during long yoga nidra sessions. I always found that approach somewhat militant, but I was up for it because I could "power" through it. I was bringing a masculine edge to my practice. Not exactly the essence of non-doing! Here are Uma's recommendations:

> I observe that a truly well-supported and comfortable experience of yoga nidra can be a receiving of nurture and nourishment, an encounter with the healing power of the deep feminine. Usually each Nidra Nest includes a couple of yoga mats or a padded mat; a couple of pillows or cushions; several bolsters for the knees; mini-bolsters for the neck and arms; and a number of warm, fluffy blankets. Eye

pillows are also on offer, and sometimes weighted blankets or sand-bags to soothe and calm the nervous system.[1]

I immediately began to reframe how I was setting up my practices and what suggestions I offered my students for setup. I supported students in creating the most luxurious throne for resting. Here is what I encountered: resistance. Resistance to deeply relaxing. Most students felt their existing setup was "good enough." But during teacher training, when co-teacher Chanti Tacoronte-Perez and I asked the same students to set up another student, they spared no indulgence in the setup. They talked with the student to make sure they were beyond comfortable, warm enough, and felt supported. Sometimes it is easier to give someone else that extra dose of love that we are not willing to give ourselves. Imagine how animals in nature will forage for anything and everything to create a nest of comfort and protection for their young. This is the kind of care and devotion you can have for your own setup. This is also a good time to review those notes from your Body Awareness Exercise to remind yourself of where you need extra support.

SETTING UP YOUR NEST

The practice of yoga nidra is passive and receptive; you are preparing yourself to be held unconditionally. It's not a time to skimp on yourself. When you are creating your yoga nidra nest, imagine that you are preparing it for your most beloved one.

Imagine that you are a king or queen, and you are creating a resting throne for yourself or a beloved. Your nest is a divine resting place. It should feel safe and comfortable, and of course, that feels different for each of us. Give yourself permission to experiment and create your own unique setup.

FIVE NEST SETUPS TO TRY

Here are a few suggestions for preparing your nest. Feel free to explore on your own, be creative, and find what works best for you.

1. The Sacred Abode

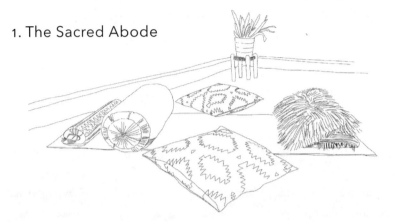

Make your nest the most comfortable place by supporting your back, ankles, head, arms, and all of your joints with props. Feel complete support. Make sure you are not too warm, which may make you fall asleep.

2. Side-Lying

Can be supportive for pregnant women (after the second trimester) or anyone with back issues.

Practice this lying on your left side and place a bolster between your knees, a pillow under your head, and use blankets to support any other part of your body that may need it—for example, feet or bony parts of the body that are resting on the floor.

3. The Recliner

Useful for those who have a tendency
to fall asleep, cough, or snore.

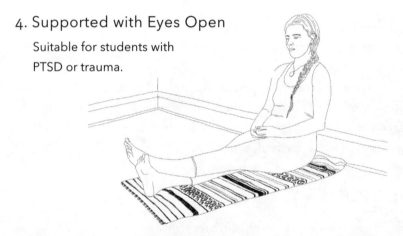

Set up your props so your head is elevated above your heart and your knees are supported. Imagine you are sitting back in a reclining chair and let the props support you. If you are a wheelchair user, blankets and props can be added to assist you in finding the most comfort.

4. Supported with Eyes Open

Suitable for students with
PTSD or trauma.

Sit leaning against a wall and facing the door. Your eyes can remain open or half-open, and your legs can be crossed. Using blankets is desired to create a cushion between your back and the wall.

5. Makarasana (Crocodile Pose)

May be supportive for students with back pain.
Not advisable for pregnant women.

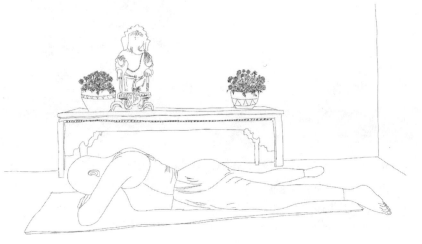

Lie on your belly. Fold your arms so one arm is resting on top of the other, and let your forehead rest on your arms. Your legs are apart with either your feet apart or heels apart and toes touching—whichever is more comfortable for you. This posture helps to support diaphragmatic breathing and allows you to access a state of relaxation as you observe the movement of the diaphragm. This posture and diaphragmatic breath awareness is considered an important preparation to accessing effortless breathing.

PROP IDEAS

Here are a few things you may want to have on hand for your practice that can help support you in creating a comfortable nest for yourself or your students. Many of these items can be found around the house.

BLANKETS AND LARGE BEACH TOWELS. You'll want something with which to cover yourself and to support your joints. It can be one large, cozy blanket and smaller blankets or towels to support your cervical spine, Achilles tendons, or arms.

WEIGHTED BLANKET. This was mentioned before, and it's a powerful tool. According to research published in the journal *Occupational Therapy in Mental Health*, weighted blankets lowered blood pressure and pulse rates and reduced anxiety for 63 percent of study participants. Check with your doctor to see if a weighted blanket might be right for you. It makes some people feel too constrained, so please test one before making the investment or using it in practice.

LIGHT SCARF OR LIGHT EYE PILLOW. Covering your eyes can assist you in turning your awareness inward. A light scarf works, or you may want a light eye pillow (After a while, a heavy eye pillow can become uncomfortable.) I have found one that is 6″ × 2½″ with a seam down the center to be the most comfortable. If it doesn't feel safe or comfortable for you to close your eyes, you can keep them open.

SILK CAMPING BAG LINER. You'll want to stay covered, especially if you are practicing outside where there may be bugs. Silk helps to regulate body temperature, warming you up in colder weather and cooling you off when it's hot, so it's excellent in any outdoor or indoor temperature. It's a permanent part of my yoga nidra nest setup.

YOGA BOLSTER, PILLOWS, OR COUCH CUSHIONS. You'll need padding to prop up your body for more support. There is no need to buy fancy yoga props when you probably have a lot of these supportive pillows lying around the house.

SOCKS. If you tend to have cold feet, you may want a pair of socks. (Tip: If I am feeling fatigued prior to practice, I don't wear socks—I use that little bit of cold to keep me alert during practice and not too cozy!)

HAND PILLOWS. You can place heavier, sandbag-style eye pillows on your hands. Some people feel that this helps to deepen their relaxation. I've seen them for sale on sites like Etsy.

SUBSTITUTIONS. If you are incarcerated or someplace where props and items found in homes are not available, rolling up a T-shirt, sweatpants, or socks can add extra support under your head or lower back. Using books or magazines covered in towels or blankets to elevate feet or other parts of the body can also be helpful.

CREATING A YOGA NIDRA ALTAR

If you feel inspired to add a yoga nidra altar to your space, it's a wonderful way to stay connected to your practice.

The word *altar* originally derives from the Latin word *altus*, meaning "high." Imagine creating a space where your highest aspirations for deep rest, surrender, and transformation are reflected.

I love creating yoga nidra altars. It is a beautiful way to affirm your devotion to the practice and to open yourself to the grace of the practices and the Goddess. If you have ever done a vision board, this is the 3D version, but it requires more care and devotion. You will have to dust it and replace flowers, incense, and candles. Your daily attention to it is a reminder not to fall asleep to your life, but to remain awake and aware. With just the few moments each day you take time to be present at your altar, it can become a portal toward awakening you to your truth.

The altar is also a way for you to remember that you are opening yourself to the grace of the state of consciousness that is yoga nidra and all the healing, wisdom, and deep rest that it can reveal to you. Ultimately this is an altar to You, to the part of you that holds the highest vibrations of healing, knowledge, and love, that is often clouded by fear, doubt, confusion, and exhaustion. It is a way for you to remember that you are committed to your practice. And if the only thing you can do during the day is to spend a moment at the altar, lighting a candle, remembering how you felt during your most profound experience of yoga nidra, and repeating one of the sankalpas to yourself quietly three times, that can be enough to keep weaving the thread of practice through your day.

Ideas for Your Altar

Keep your altar free of clutter. Place it somewhere where you can see it every day—on a nightstand next to your bed is a great idea. Remember, these are suggestions, so be creative with what and how you create an altar; the essential thing is that it has meaning to you and that you feel inspired to visit it every day.

SYMBOL OF SURRENDER. The first thing to do to prepare your altar is to review your self-inquiry answers in chapter 3 (page 71), mainly those that reflect your thoughts about deserving rest. Recall any other resistance to rest and relaxation that might have shown up. What do you need to overcome to allow yourself the depth of rest, healing, and self-care that yoga nidra can provide? Write or draw what you need to let go of to move toward a new depth of surrender on a small piece of paper and frame it. You might try something like this:

I commit to releasing _____. I deserve
deep rest and relaxation. It is my birthright. I practice to realize my
true nature and have it manifest in my life as _____.

MEMORIAL TO ANCESTORS. Add the images or names of ancestors or those who are helpful guides for you and are close to your heart.

SACRED INSPIRATION. What would you do if you were truly rested? How would your power manifest and express itself? Place something that reminds you of how you envision truly thriving on your altar.

MEMENTOS FROM PEACEFUL PLACES. Find pictures, art, or poetry that remind you of the places that bring you the most peace. Search for pictures of places that you hope to visit and place them on your altar.

INVOCATION TO THE GODDESS YOGA NIDRA. If the concept of Yoga Nidra as a goddess resonates with you, you can write a poem, find images that invoke her presence, or learn the verse from the Devi Suktam or verse 10 from the Ratri Suktum. You might find additional inspiration about goddesses from other cultures, such as Mawu from Yoruba culture or the Greek goddess Selene, that share similar moonlike nurturing qualities.

THE FIVE ELEMENTS. Most altars have representations of the five elements. As you begin to move through the practices, especially the nature-amplification practices, you may be inspired by your experiences to add things from those environments or to create new affirmations or poetry that remind you of your experiences. If you would like to have the elements represented on your altar, here are some ideas:

- *Earth.* Fresh flowers, rocks, soil. The earth element reminds us of the impermanence of life, that we will all return to the earth one day. Earth connects to the wisdom that we are supported by the beauty of this incredibly generous and abundant planet that offers us so many treasures. The earth element can connect you to gratitude for this support and is a wonderful way to honor the earth as our oldest ancestor. You may also be inspired to make an offering back to the earth to show your gratitude.

- *Fire.* A candle or flame; when fire itself is not appropriate, a crystal such as citrine, amber, carnelian, ruby, sunstone, or fire opal. Fire represents transformation and the power of our practices to reveal knowledge that burns away our ignorance. Fire allows us to have gratitude for the heat and friction that our practices bring to our lives and the inner radiance that is revealed as a result.
- *Water.* A water vessel. Water represents purification and grace. It allows us to remember that life ebbs and flows. Water can connect us to gratitude for the ability to flow; to be creative; and to find ways to adapt, adjust, and move through our environments with a balance of ease, persistence, or power as needed.
- *Air.* Incense, a feather. Air is one of the most subtle elements that we can perceive. The five winds known as the *prana vayus* move throughout the body, keeping us both mentally and physically integrated and our systems circulating. We are reminded of our birthright of breath, and we can honor all those who are no longer breathing when we offer gratitude to the air element.
- *Ether.* A bell. Ether represents the vibration of AUM that can purify the space around us. Ether, or space, is the element that all other elements fill. We can offer gratitude for ether as it holds our prayers and the unseen and provides a container of space for us to expand into as we grow and transform spiritually.

ANYTHING ELSE THAT INSPIRES YOU. This altar is your creation and should feel specific to what inspires devotion in you. You can include any images, poems, or artwork that remind you that you are supported and loved unconditionally.

YOGA NIDRA VERSUS SLEEP FLOW

As you prepare for yoga nidra, consider your intentions in the practice. If you're concerned that lying down and turning inward can make you fall asleep, it might. We have already talked about how closely this practice can resemble sleep, with the exception of consciousness remaining awake and aware. Over the years, many of the students who have attended my workshops have told me they are using yoga nidra practice to go to sleep. It makes sense that this practice, which provides such deep relaxation and nurturing, can lull you to sleep. Yet one of the benefits of yoga nidra practice is that it can help you to *wake up* to the unseen realms of life and reality, to help you transcend attachment to that which is impermanent, and to foster your relationship with that which is eternal.

If you are experiencing insomnia, I am sure you could care less about a relationship with the eternal. You desperately want to get some much-needed rest! We all know that you cannot "catch up" on sleep, so that means that the sleep or rest you do get has to be deep and high quality. Deep relaxation practices can help. It's all about intention.

As a yoga nidra practitioner, one of the most important things to do when you have insomnia is to create a delineation between your yoga nidra practice and the practice you use to fall asleep. I suggest approaching yoga nidra as a personally transformative practice that also provides you with deep transformative rest. When you are doing a practice to try to fall asleep, think of those practices as your "Sleep Flow." Approach them with the same reverence and devotion as you would your yoga practice. I like the word *flow* instead of *practice* because it feels effortless and differentiates the desired result of the practice, which in this case would be sleep. Taking a "practice" to bed with you feels like something else you have to *do*. Use your Sleep Flow as a way to fall in love with the idea of sleep, as opposed to treating it as an enemy or a lover who has abandoned you. Your yoga nidra practice and the bedtime rituals can connect you to the power of recognizing the liminal space just before you go to sleep and may be helpful in assisting you in learning how to fall asleep.

Where and When to Practice Your Sleep Flow

To further separate your Sleep Flow from your yoga nidra practice, avoid using your bed as a place to practice yoga nidra as a spiritual or transformational practice. The bed is associated with sleep—or perhaps the frustration of not being able to sleep. Either way, there is an energy in your bed that has accumulated over time. And since you usually have no way of knowing what that energy is, try practicing yoga nidra in a separate space with your yoga nidra nest setup. You wouldn't take your yoga mat into bed and sleep on it, so don't create a nest on the same bed that you sleep in at night if at all possible. If it's unavoidable, try switching out the blankets and pillows that you use during nidra, so they are not the same ones you use at night. Over time, the shawl, eye pillows, and items in your nest will carry the energy of Nidra Shakti, which will empower your spiritual practice of yoga nidra and the ability to stay awake and aware during practice.

Your bed and bedroom should serve one purpose—to provide the most nurturing, safe, dark, womblike space of peace and healing for you to sleep and dream. Blue light is not your friend. Do everything you can to eradicate it from your sleeping space. Remove your TV and all electronic devices from your bedroom. If it's not possible to move the TV, cover it with a tapestry when it is not in use and use light-blocking LED covers for your cable box and similar devices. This is where you'll practice your Sleep Flow when you get into bed at night. So even though some of the steps may feel familiar, you will have the intention to fall asleep.

Try to practice yoga nidra in the morning, sometime before noon, so it's not too close to bedtime. Yoga nidra is essential for staying rested when you have insomnia. Your Sleep Flow will only be for nighttime when you are ready for bed.

There are a few more things you can do to help your sleep hygiene:

· Watch the sunset or look into the sky when the sun is going down, even if you can't see the sun setting.
· Begin to do things that indicate you are winding down for the day. Find your own transition routine to signal to your body that it's time to move toward sleep. You might try some restorative poses.
· Avoid eating too late at night.

- Take a warm bath 90 minutes before bedtime. (It will help change your body's core temperature.)
- Practice silence 30 minutes before bed.
- Set the temperature in your bedroom to between 60°F and 67°F.
- Experiment and take notes on what works for you. If your insomnia is chronic, see a specialist or join a sleep study. I've listed some places to look in the "Recommended Resources" section.
- Consider taking an herb tonic to help you sleep. The following Ayurvedic tonic, from teacher Laura Plumb, is my all-time favorite and gives me a deep sleep every time.

Deep Sleep Tonic

Courtesy of Ayurvedic practitioner Laura Plumb

10 almonds, soaked for 8 hours and then skinned*
1 cup whole milk (dairy, almond, or rice)
2 teaspoons ghee
4–5 dates, preferably medjool
8 black peppercorns
½ teaspoon cardamom
½ teaspoon cinnamon
Pinch each cumin, turmeric, and nutmeg

Liquefy all the ingredients in a blender until the mixture reaches a smooth consistency. Pour into a pot on the stove and bring it to a very gentle boil. Stir and serve.

*If you haven't presoaked the almonds, simply blanche them in boiling water for 1 minute. Drain and run under cold water, then remove and discard their skins.

· Sleep Flow ·

Inspired by the teaching of Swami Rama

[5 minutes]

When you are ready to do your Sleep Flow to fall asleep, take a moment to create an intention:

I welcome the grace of deep sleep.
May I be rested, rejuvenated, and healed by my sleep.

---

1. Lie down in Makarasana (Crocodile Pose, page 183).
2. Inhale for 4 counts; exhale for 8 counts. Focus your awareness on the rise and fall of your belly. Notice the breath. Do not force your breathing, just watch the flow, feel the breath becoming effortless, silent, even, and smooth like warm oil being poured from a pitcher. Feel breath moving into your sides and your back. (2 minutes)
3. Roll to your right side. Feel as though you are breathing only through your left nostril and that the whole left side of your body is breathing. Inhale for 4 counts; exhale for 8 counts. (2 minutes)
4. Roll to your left side. Feel as though the entire right side of your body is breathing. Notice the flow of your natural breath with each inhalation. Continue to feel as though the whole right side is breathing. (2 minutes)
5. Come to rest on your back and just watch your navel rising and falling as you inhale for 4 counts and exhale for 8 counts. (18 times) Feel the body becoming heavier and heavier with each exhalation. Let your body go into the support of the bed, trusting you are held. Feel the body releasing and remember your intention, *May I be rested, rejuvenated, and healed by my sleep.* Repeat it to yourself 3–9 times.

6. See a full moon resting at your throat center. (3 minutes)
7. Let your awareness move to your heart center, the center of deep sleep. (3 minutes)
8. Let go and surrender into the spaciousness of the heart as you fall asleep.

· PART 3 ·

Yoga Nidra Practices

THIS PART OF THE BOOK presents several practices to help guide and prepare you to receive the state and grace of yoga nidra. Each practice includes poses, pranayama practices, and mantras that can also help you get the most out of the practices of deep relaxation. You can experiment with these pre-practices to see which of them are most helpful to you. The deep relaxation practices are designed to move you from the grossest layer of your being to the most subtle, starting with Practice One, which focuses on the relaxation of the physical body, and progressing to Practice Six, which focuses on true freedom. Each of the deep relaxation practices is also available as an audio recording to help guide you. Visit www.Shambhala.com/RadiantRestPractices to access them.

Spend time with these practices. Create a forty-day commitment to *sadhana* (dedicated practice) and use the thread of the Householder's Flow to keep the practices alive and awake within you when you don't have time to lie down for a longer practice.

Every time you do one of these practices, you will learn more about yourself: how your breath changes when you are relaxed, which position is most comfortable, which props you really need, where you are holding tension, which recurring thoughts prevent you from relaxing, and what it feels like to "drop in deeply." The fruit of all your previous practices is invaluable and will inform your next practice. Taking time to keep a journal will activate your *smirti shakti* (power of retention and memory) and allow you to develop more self-knowledge.

If you are a teacher, the key is to embody each practice before you teach it. Use the practices in this book to prepare yourself to take a live yoga nidra training course with a skilled instructor.

Consistent practice, whether you are a teacher or a seeker, will help you awaken to your deepest truth and knowing. It is with that wish that I offer these practices to you.

· 6 ·

Practice One
Grounding and Stability

THIS PRACTICE INVITES you to explore the grossest element, earth, which is associated with your physical body, the annamaya kosha. Through this practice, you'll develop your ability to release held tension and constriction and connect with the earth's grounding vibration.

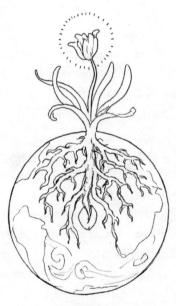

BENEFITS

Presence

Sense of the physical body in space

Cultivation of stillness

Awareness of sensations of the physical body

PRACTICE THIS . . .

- Any time you are experiencing feelings of being ungrounded, scattered, or overwhelmed.
- During or right after lengthy travel to help balance feelings of constant movement.
- As a daily practice to begin your day.

TEACH THIS . . .

- As a substitute for Savasana with music.
- If you're adding this as a deep relaxation practice after an asana class, allow your students to receive a few minutes of spacious silence and perhaps time to journal, which will assist them in processing and assimilating the depth of their practice.

It's not uncommon these days to feel life is just go, go, go without any time to pause and rest. Even during times when we have to stay at home, we can feel pressure to produce, to be on social media, or to create lists of all the things we need to get done. It is so hard to slow down, even when we get messages from the body that it's time to stop. This grounding practice helps balance that feeling of constant movement. It will help you gain a deeper understanding of your physical body and how you relate to the space around you. It will also allow you to develop *asana shakti*, which the Vedic teacher

David Frawley defines as "the power to rest comfortably in a single posture without internal friction where we easily forget body consciousness and naturally move within."[1] With consistent practice, you will become more aware of where you unconsciously hold tension in your body. This will deepen your understanding of the physical body as the annamaya kosha (food sheath), the grossest and densest part of the subtle body and the outermost of the nesting dolls that hold your Divine light.

PREPARING FOR DEEP RELAXATION

Moving the body, breath, and prana are great ways to prepare the body for rest. These preparatory practices are optional. When you can, take the time for them and notice how they support and enhance your experience.

Self-Massage

In Ayurveda, the practice of massaging your body with oil (*abhyanga*) is a grounding daily ritual. Try oils such as avocado or sesame oil to massage your body with a loving touch. You can warm your oil and rub it in using circular strokes around your joints and long, sweeping strokes on your arms and legs; all strokes should move toward the heart.

Poses

Spend a few minutes in one or two of the following poses while remaining aware of your breath:

Makarasana (Crocodile Pose, page 183)
Apanasana (Knees-to-Chest Pose, page 181)
Balasana (Child's Pose, page 181)
Paschimottanasana (Seated Forward Bend, page 183)
Malasana (Garland Pose, page 182)

Pranayama

1:2 Breathing (page 191) *5 minutes*

Apana Vayu (Downward-Moving Air) Meditation[2] (page 192) *3 minutes*

Sankalpa

I honor and acknowledge my body as a sacred vessel that houses my inner light. I invite deep rest into every cell of my being. I trust that I deserve to be supported, nurtured, and held unconditionally. I *know* the earth can hold me.

Mantra

Sit in your meditation posture, bring your attention to the base of your spine, and feel your connection to the earth. Mentally or verbally chant the mantras. *5 minutes*

GAM (*gum*), LAM (*lum*)

· Grounding Deep Relaxation Practice ·
[15–20 minutes]

Come into your yoga nidra nest. Make sure your body is comfortable and supported by any pillows, blankets, or other props you need. Set your timer for 15 to 20 minutes. If you have more space in your schedule, you may choose not to use a timer.

If you feel comfortable closing your eyes, do so; if not, leave them gently open, gazing softly. Take three deep breaths: inhaling and filling your lungs, exhaling and emptying your lungs with a deep sigh out. Be aware of your breath, each time you exhale, feel a wave of relaxation sweep through your body as you release and let go. (10 breaths)

Invite stillness into your body. Be aware of the space your body is occupying. (2 minutes) Imagine that you are drawing a circle of protection around your body. This circle can be made of anything you wish: fire, Divine light, your favorite flowers, fresh soil, limbs of trees, or a wall of clay. Whatever calls to you, establish this circle of protection around yourself. See and feel yourself inside the circle. (1 minute)

As you become more still, begin to feel the breath as it enters your nostrils. Feel it travel into your lungs, where it dissolves. Then follow its path all the way to somewhere outside your body, where it dissolves again. You are not controlling the breath. You are merely watching it move in and out of your body. Feel your navel rise and fall as you breathe in and out. (2 minutes)

Feel yourself lying on the earth. Slowly scan through your body and become aware of how you are holding it. You may recall the body parts that felt constricted during your earlier body awareness exercise. Feel free to let your body adjust for one more layer of comfort. (2 minutes)

Let your awareness move toward sound, noticing all the sounds around you without judgment. Allow your awareness to move from sound to sound to sound. Let all the sounds be there. You are on the inside of the circle; the sounds are on its circumference. (1 minute) Remember your sankalpa:

I honor and acknowledge my body as a sacred vessel that houses my inner light. I invite deep rest into every cell of my being. I trust that I deserve to be supported, nurtured, and held unconditionally. I *know* the earth can hold me.

Notice the parts of your body that are touching the floor. Begin at your feet and scan upward. Feel your heels touching the floor and silently repeat the mantra LAM (*lum*). Feel the next point where your body contacts the floor and repeat LAM. Continue all the way until you get to the top of your head:

Calves and the floor, LAM
Backs of your thighs and the floor, LAM
Buttocks and the floor, LAM
Parts of your spine touching the floor, LAM
Shoulder blades and the floor, LAM
Back of your head and the floor, LAM

Feel all of these body parts becoming heavier as you repeat the mantra LAM. Notice your body breathing. As it receives an inhalation, sense the earth rising up to hold and cradle you. It's as though the involuntary act of inhaling is calling the earth toward you.

As your body exhales, ask it to surrender into the earth. Every in-breath invites the earth to support you even more. Every out-breath is a trusting acceptance that you deserve to be held. Begin with the number 27 and begin to count backward:

Inhale, 27; exhale, 27.
Inhale, 26; exhale, 26.

Each time you exhale, a layer of constriction and tension is released from your body and mind. By the time you get to zero, the body and mind are completely free. If you lose your place when counting, start again from 27. Once you get to zero, feel the earth holding you unconditionally. (3 minutes) Feel your body and the earth breathing as one. (5 minutes)

Now begin to transition out of the practice, noticing everything during this transition. Welcome yourself back. Notice the breath. Notice your body. Notice the earth beneath you. Begin to deepen your breath. (1–2 minutes)

Slowly roll to your right side and sit up. Spend 3 minutes freewriting anything that comes to mind. Then answer the self-inquiry questions that follow.

SELF-INQUIRY

Directly after your deep relaxation practice, allow yourself 10 to 15 minutes to answer these questions. Write as fast as you can. Don't worry about your grammar or sentence structure. Feel as though the flame at the altar of your heart is guiding your hand. You may answer the questions in words, poetry, dance, drawing, or painting. Just let it flow. As you continue with this practice, come back to these questions periodically and answer them again.

1. What activities make you feel most grounded?
2. Do you trust that you have support?
3. How have you rejected others' desire to support you in the past? Why?
4. Describe a time when you felt truly supported and held. If you cannot connect to such a time, write about what you imagine it feeling like.
5. Name one thing that you can stop doing today that causes you to feel a lack of stability.

DAILY PRACTICES

Choose at least one of the following shorter practices on days when you don't have time for deep relaxation and self-inquiry.

Bedtime Ritual: I Am Held *10 minutes*

As you prepare to sleep, take care to feel your feet on the ground before getting into bed. Slide into bed leading with your left foot.

Lie on your belly in Makarasana (Crocodile Pose, page 183). As you inhale and exhale, bring your awareness to your belly, and feel your navel expanding on the in-breath and contracting on the out-breath. As you become more aware of your breath, begin to inhale for a count of 3 and exhale for a count of 6. If your breath capacity is greater, it may feel more comfortable to increase the count to 4 or 5 and then exhale for twice as long. (10 minutes)

Turn over and prepare for sleep, finding a comfortable sleeping position. Feel your body on the bed, supported and comfortable. Notice where you do not feel supported and create more support by adjusting your pillows, placing one between your legs or wrapping your arms around a pillow if needed. When you feel at ease, bring awareness to your heart. Keeping your awareness there, take a deep breath and exhale with an audible sweet and gentle sigh. (9 times)

Keep your awareness at your heart. Remember your gratitude toward the earth for its stability, strength, and capacity to hold you. Repeat to yourself, *I am supported; I am held.* (3 times)

Keeping your awareness at your heart, allow yourself to drift off to sleep.

Wake-Up Ritual: I Am Supported *2–5 minutes*

As you notice yourself transitioning back to wakefulness, begin to feel the liminal space between sleeping and waking. Remember the thread of your nighttime affirmation: *I am supported; I am held.* Continue to repeat this silently to yourself.

Bring your awareness to your heart center and slowly breathe more deeply, allowing your limbs to move and stretch. Exit the bed with your right foot first, feel your connection to the earth, and then with full presence feel both feet connect with the earth. Pause and feel the ground beneath you.

Take time to write down a few ways that you feel supported and also note where you could use more support or ask for assistance. Remember the affirmation throughout your day.

Nature-Amplification Practice: Earth Vibration *15 minutes*

Find a space outdoors to do this practice—preferably a grassy park or backyard or a beach, somewhere you feel safe that is relatively quiet and free of insects. Set your timer for 15 minutes, or longer if you have time.

Lie on the ground. Ask the earth to support you and offer your gratitude. If you are on the beach (my favorite place to practice this), dig yourself into the sand. Or depending on where you are, you can nestle in the grass or lie on a flat rock. Any place where you are in contact with the ground will work.

Arrange yourself so you are fully supported in every way. For example, build the ultimate support in the sand for your heels, buttocks, lower back, and neck. If you are lying on the ground, bring a blanket or pillow if desired. I often do this practice spontaneously without any props on hand. Wherever you are, get comfortable.

Take three deep breaths in through your nose and out through your mouth with a deep sigh. Let your breath be natural. Just notice it. (1 minute)

Feel yourself resting on the earth. Repeat to yourself, *Dear Earth, please hold me. I trust that you can hold me and everything that I am holding.* (3 times)

Feel and sense everything around you: the surface you are lying on, the breeze on your skin, the warmth of the sun, or the coolness of the evening air. Let the noises around you fade into the distance as you listen to your breath flowing in and out. Notice the temperature of the earth beneath you.

Notice how you are supported and be still. The more still you become, the more you will observe a gentle vibration coming from the earth. Feel that vibration. Now feel your body. Now back to the vibration.

As you inhale, feel that you are drawing in this vibration through every pore of your body; as you exhale, sense that you are letting go of toxins, worry, and stress through those same pores. Imagine that everything you release is being composted back into the earth. Remember that the earth can hold you. (2 minutes)

Feel the vibration of the earth and your body as the two vibrations merge to become one. Rest. Let yourself be held. Once your timer goes off, just come up to sitting. Sit in silence. In your own way, offer gratitude to the earth. (1 minute)

Open your eyes and spend 3 to 10 minutes freewriting.

· 7 ·

Practice Two

Waves of AUM

THESE PRACTICES CONNECT you with the fluid, purifying, nurturing quality of an energy that flows like water. They can help you to establish your ability to ride the ebb and flow of life. The deep relaxation practice has been taught in many variations and originates with wisdom from texts such as the Saura-purana, which refer to drawing prana to eighteen spots in the body as a pratyahara practice.[1] This practice highlights the process of dissolution as you gradually dissolve parts of the body and the elements associated with those parts of the body (see page 116).

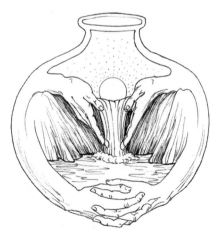

BENEFITS

Energetic reset
Sense of bodily ease and freedom
Detachment from negative emotions
Transformation and expansion
Purification

PRACTICE THIS . . .

· Any time you feel the desire for an energetic reset.
· If you have been hanging out in a toxic environment.
· To release anxiety and stress.
· To deepen your experience of meditation and yoga nidra.
· Right before a creative exercise such as journaling, painting, or writing poetry.

TEACH THIS . . .

· To enhance sensitivity to prana and pranamaya kosha.
· To develop pratyahara, which allows you to return to your true nature.
· To explore the practice of dissolution (laya yoga).

If you have been spending time in a toxic environment (a space where there has been negativity, a fight, or just a bad attitude) and want to fill yourself with fresh energy or return back to the source of peace within you, these are your tools. They will help you to develop a sense of ease and may help you to detach from negative emotions. Both the shusumna meditation and the deep relaxation practices will help sensitize you to prana and pranamaya kosha. The deep relaxation is also a pratyahara practice in the fullest sense, asking us to withdraw our senses and dissolve awareness of our body parts. This practice also allows us to touch the transitional space between our inner personal space (aura) and the outer space by bringing awareness to the space twelve inches above the crown of our head known as *dvadashanta*. If you are feeling ungrounded or are a beginner in this practice, skip the last step of going to twelve inches above the crown and instead follow prana from the third eye to the crown. Take a moment to review the illustration on page 116 for reference.[2]

With consistency, these will support your ability to remain steady in the midst of change while watching the ebb and flow of life with more discernment, detachment, and curiosity.

PREPARING FOR DEEP RELAXATION

Moving the body, breath, and prana are great ways to prepare the body for rest. These preparatory practices are optional. When you can, take the time for them and notice how they support and enhance your experience.

Poses

Spend a few minutes moving in and out of one or two of the following poses, coordinating your movements with your breath:

Hip Circles in Table-Top Position (page 182)
Figure Eights in Table-Top Position (page 182)

Pranayama

Shusumna Meditation (page 192) *10 minutes*

Sankalpa

My in-breath is an invitation for vital energy to support and nourish me. My out-breath is the acknowledgment of my longing to be free. My breath reaches far and wide. I allow the universe to hold me. I am cleansed by her waves of love. I am free.

Mantra

Sit in your meditation posture, visualize the area of the sacrum, pelvic center, or womb. Mentally or verbally chant the mantras. *5 minutes*

VAM (*vum*), AUM

VAM is the mantra for water and the second chakra. AUM is the mantra that represents the whole of the universe and the states of consciousness; it is the seed sound of energy and vitality.

· Deep Relaxation Practice: Waves of AUM ·
[30–40 minutes]

Come into your yoga nidra nest, lying on your back, lying on your side, or sitting against the wall. Once you are in your comfortable position, in your own way, draw a circle of protection around your body. (1 minute)

Let your awareness move toward sound, noticing all of the sounds around you without judgment or inquiry. Allow your awareness to move from sound to sound to sound. (1 minute) Let all the sounds be there. You are on the inside of the circle; all the sounds become distant on the outside of the circle. (1 minute) Notice your breath as your navel moves up as you inhale and down as you exhale. (2 minutes)

Feel the breath come into your body from your nostrils and move to the crown of your head. As you exhale, feel the breath move from the crown of your head to the tip of your toes. Follow the inhalation back up to the top of your head.

Count these breaths backward from 10 to zero. You are letting go of constriction and tension in the body and mind with each out-breath. Stay focused on counting. Exhale, 10; inhale, 10; exhale, 9; inhale, 9; and so on. If you lose your place, start back at 10. Once you finish counting, just notice the breath. (1 minute)

Follow the flow of your next exhalation. Feel it move from the crown of your head down the center of your body and out between your legs, continuing through the space between your feet. Feel your next inhalation move up between your feet and through the center of your body to the crown of your head.

On the next exhalation, silently repeat or feel the vibration of AAAUUUMMM moving with the breath as it flows from the crown of your head, down the center of your body, and out through the space between your feet. Feel that sound of AUM as it rides on the breath flowing all the way to the edge of your yoga mat.

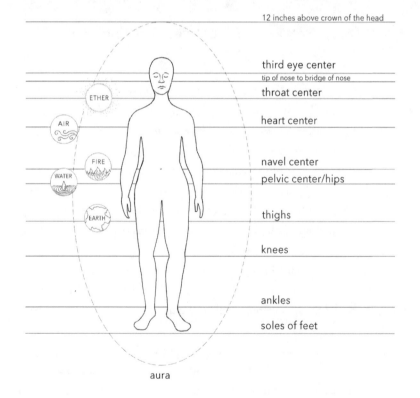

12 inches above crown of the head

third eye center

tip of nose to bridge of nose

throat center

heart center

navel center

pelvic center/hips

thighs

knees

ankles

soles of feet

ETHER

AIR

FIRE

WATER

EARTH

aura

As you inhale AUM, feel as though you are pulling the breath and the vibration of AUM all the way from the edge of your yoga mat between your feet, between your legs, and up your spine to the crown of your head. Let the exhalation of AUM flow all the way to the door of the room you are lying in.

As you inhale, feel the AUM breath flow back to the crown of your head. Every exhalation moves progressively farther and wider out into space. Feel the AUM exhalation flow out to your favorite tree, and inhale AUM back up to the crown of your head. (5 times) Exhale AUM and let it flow out to the sky; inhale it back up to the crown of your head. (5 times)

Feel the AUM exhalation flow to the edge of the ocean and then inhale back to the crown of your head. (5 times)

The AUM breath flows all the way to the land on the other side of the ocean and then back to the crown of your head. (5 times)

The AUM breath flows to the moon and then flows back to the crown of your head. (5 times)

The AUM breath flows all the way to the brightest star and back to the crown of your head. (5 times)

The AUM breath travels all the way to the farthest reaches of the universe and returns to the top of your head. (5 times)

Rest in stillness and silence, experiencing the sound of AUM vibrating through your body and feeling the flow of prana (vital life force). Bring your awareness to the soles of your feet. Feel that vibration of AUM, prana, or presence as a wave that rides on the breath. Rest in the vibration of AUM.[3] Remember your sankalpa:

My in-breath is an invitation for vital energy to support and
nourish me. My out-breath is the acknowledgment of my longing
to be free. My breath reaches far and wide. I allow the universe
to hold me. I am cleansed by her waves of love. I am free.

Inhale and exhale, feeling that prana or a presence is riding on the breath. (1 minute) Inhale and feel that vibration or presence traveling from the soles of your feet all the way to the crown of your head. As you exhale, the wave of prana moves back down to the soles of your feet. (3 minutes)

Let your next breath travel from your ankles to the top of your head and back down to your ankles. (3 minutes) Feel waves of prana flow from the middle of your calves to the top of your head and back to the middle of your calves. (2 minutes) Feel prana move from your knees to the top of your head and back to your knees. (2 minutes)

Follow prana from your hips to the crown of your head and back to your hips. (1 minute) Follow prana from your pelvic center to the crown of your head. (1 minute)

Watch prana and presence move from your navel center to the crown of your head and back to your navel. (1 minute) Feel prana move from your heart center to the crown of your head and back to your heart center. (1 minute) Feel prana flow from your throat center to the crown of your head and back to your throat center. (1 minute)

Watch prana move from the root of your tongue to the crown of your head and back to the root of your tongue. (1 minute)

Inhale and sense prana moving from the tip of your nose to the bridge of your nose and back to the tip.[4] (2 minutes)

Inhale and sense presence moving from your third eye center to a space twelve inches above your head and back to your third eye. (5 minutes)

Rest in spacious awareness. (3–5 minutes)

Let awareness rest at each of the energy centers in your body and feel the vibration of AUM at each energy center:

Third eye	Navel center
Throat center	Pelvic center
Heart center	Base of the spine

As you end the practice, place your fingertips on the ground, feeling the connection as though a grounding cord is connecting you to the earth. Welcome yourself back. Breathe in and out deeply. (3 times) Roll to your side and then slowly sit up. Spend 5 minutes freewriting.

SELF-INQUIRY

Directly after your deep relaxation practice, allow yourself 10 to 15 minutes to answer the following questions. Write as fast as you can. Don't worry about your grammar or sentence structure. Feel as though your heart is guiding your hand. You may answer the questions in words, poetry, dance, drawing, or painting. Just let it flow. As you continue with this practice, come back to these questions periodically and answer them again.

1. What mind-set is most helpful for you to weather life's storms?
2. What keeps you from experiencing this mind-set in times of tumult? What do you need to remember?
3. What possible changes in life are you most fearful of?
4. Which of the changes are inevitable? How can you make peace with them and mindfully prepare for their arrival?

DAILY PRACTICES

Choose at least one of the following shorter practices on days when you don't have time for deep relaxation and self-inquiry.

Bedtime Ritual: Moon Bath and Breath *5–10 minutes*

This practice can be done indoors or outdoors under the light of the full moon, or you can just imagine a full moon. If you have trouble visualizing, take a look at a few images of the moon prior to practicing.

Sit quietly right before bedtime. Visualize the moon directly above your head—a full, bright moon. See, sense, or feel that light is radiating from this full moon. For a few moments, breathe through both nostrils. Without trying to control or shape the breath, just watch it flow in and out. Now notice that one of your nostrils is more open than the other. The breath feels stronger in one nostril. Feel as though you can breathe just through the dominant nostril.

Breathe just through the dominant nostril, in and out through the same nostril. (1 minute) Now if it's not there already, move your awareness to your left nostril. Inhale, feeling the vapors of the moon entering the left nostril and exiting the right nostril as you exhale. Feel this moonlight creating a nurturing, refreshing, and calm feeling.

Inhale through the left nostril for four counts and exhale through the right for eight counts. (3 minutes)

Remember the moon directly above your head. Feel as though the nectar of the moon is raining down on you like a shower of moonlit raindrops. Feel it invoking a sense of peace and tranquility as it is absorbed into every cell of your body. Gently massage your body with light, loving stokes, as if you are massaging this healing nectar into your skin. Massage your face, arms, legs, and chest. Lie down to sleep with a vision of the moon resting in your throat center.

Wake-Up Ritual: Radiant Moon Wake-Up *3 minutes*

As you feel yourself becoming conscious, rest in the transition between sleeping and waking. Reach into the watery essence of dreamtime and notice where your consciousness is moving. Feel the liminal quality between being asleep and fully awake. Remember the healing nectar of the full moon from the night before as you feel yourself waking and coming up to sitting. Notice any thoughts and let them go, especially the ones that ask you for "just five more minutes" of sleep!

Remember your sankalpa:

> My in-breath is an invitation for vital energy to support and
> nourish me. My out-breath is the acknowledgment of my longing
> to be free. My breath reaches far and wide. I allow the universe
> to hold me. I am cleansed by her waves of love. I am free.

Feel each in-breath and out-breath. Feel yourself becoming enlivened and refreshed. Each breath brings in vitality and releases the heaviness and inertia from the night before. Remember the nectar of the moon and feel it still raining down to nurture and support you.

Begin to anoint and bless your body once again with the nectar of the moon. Imagine you are massaging it into your body lovingly but with a more rigorous touch than the night before, waking up each body part with a gentle yet firm massage. (3 minutes)

After your massage is complete, spend 5 minutes freewriting.

Nature-Amplification Practice: Elemental Activation *15–20 minutes*

Find yourself a place near a stream, ocean, or fountain, somewhere where you can hear the water moving—undulating waves, trickling, or bubbling up. Stay a safe distance away from the actual water, where you do not have to worry about an encroaching tide, but close enough that you can hear the water. If you don't have access to water right now, you can find recordings of waves online or listen to the audio version of this meditation.

Take a moment to find a comfortable, safe spot to lie down. Let all of your attention begin to follow your natural flow of breath. You are not trying to control your breath; you are merely watching yourself breathe. Watch your belly rise and fall. Silently repeat, *The body breathes in; the body breathes out*, as you observe the breath flowing in and out. (10 breaths)

Notice your body on the ground. Feel the vibration of the earth, and notice your connection to it. Take a moment to offer gratitude for the element of water. Feel the temperature of the earth beneath you. Can you sense any moisture in the air? Notice the difference between this air and the air you usually breathe.

Feel the breath as it enters your body. Feel the space that your body is occupying. Feel the quality of the air around you. Listen to the sounds of the water. (2 minutes)

Remember that your body is made up of about 60 percent water. Offer gratitude for this water and the life it gives you. Feel the fluids in your body—the saliva in your mouth, the blood in your veins. Imagine there is an upward-flowing river in your spine. Feel it flowing from the base of your spine toward the crown of your head each time you inhale. (2 minutes)

Sense the river expanding to the size of your whole body. Feel your whole body as flowing water. Notice the waves, the ebbs and flows. Notice how neither the ebb nor the flow is important; it just is. Let go and observe yourself as a body of water. (2 minutes)

Each time you breathe out, feel as though you begin to evaporate just a little, rising up as a fine mist or steam to join the clouds. (5 breaths)

See those clouds darkening and transforming into rain clouds. Visualize yourself showering down from the sky in the form of raindrops, like healing nectar watering the earth, moving through porous rock and deep into the aquifer, and then traveling up a windy passage through a fault in the earth to a bubbling stream. (2 minutes)

See yourself as a raindrop falling into the vast ocean. (2 minutes)

Feel and sense yourself as flowing water. Ride the ebbs and flows. Let go of doing. (5 minutes)

Come back to listening to the sounds of water and deepen the breath. Let it bring you fully back into your body, feeling refreshed, revitalized, and grateful.

· 8 ·

Practice Three

Deep Relaxation, Essential Activation

THIS PRACTICE ACTIVATES your vital life force and purifies the body and mind by placing mantra, light, or awareness systematically throughout the body in various *marma* points.

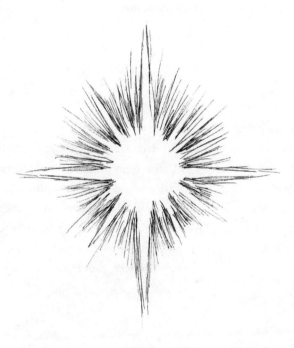

BENEFITS

Refreshing

Development of one-pointed focus

Development of inner awareness of our cosmic nature

Deep relaxation for the body and mind

Development of discipline

PRACTICE THIS . . .

· When you are feeling anxious.

· Before taking an exam.

· When you have important decisions to make.

· Any time you need a mental or physical reset.

· When your energy feels heavy or dull.

TEACH THIS . . .

· Anytime.

When in doubt, this is your go-to practice. If you are a teacher and this were the only practice you offered your students, it would be enough. Most of the students I see in my coaching practice report feeling varying levels of stress and anxiety. They are worried about work, finances, children, aging parents, or the safety of the world. They feel out of balance, deprived of creativity, and lacking in the spaciousness and resources they need to follow their dreams. They cannot turn off their minds. This practice will help you redirect your focus inward, enliven your energetic body, and settle your mind.

PREPARING FOR DEEP RELAXATION

Moving the body, breath, and prana are great ways to prepare the body for rest. These preparatory practices are optional. When you can, take the time for them and notice how they support and enhance your experience.

Poses

Spend a few minutes in one or two of the following poses or movements:

Chakravakasana flow sequence (Cat-Cow Pose, page 181) Chant AUM as you exhale.
Savasana (Corpse Pose, page 183)
Makarasana (Crocodile Pose, page 183) with Diaphragmatic Breathing (page 190)
Slow and gentle intuitive movements while breathing deeply
Breath-centric asana (any asanas performed by linking movement and breath with intention and presence)
Dancing to release tension and to express and release emotions

Pranayama

Choose any one of the following to practice, notice its effects, and make notes.

Bhramari Breath (Humming of the Bees, page 189) *9 times*

1:2 Breathing (page 191) *5 minutes*

Nadi Shodhana (Alternate Nostril Breathing, page 190) *3 minutes*

Sankalpa

May my mind be a flow of beautiful and divine resolves, filled with auspicious thoughts. (A translation of the last refrain of the Shiva Sankalpa Sukta.)

Mantra

TAN ME MANAHA SHIVA SANKALPAM ASTU

May my mind be filled with auspicious thoughts.

This mantra is a refrain from the Shiva Sankalpa Sukta. Swami Veda Bharati said that this refrain holds the benefits of the six verses that comprise the entire mantra and is perfect for those who cannot or do not have time to memorize the full mantra. The mantra as a whole invites the mind to follow a flow of thought that is in alignment with your highest purpose. (See the full mantra on page 188.)

· Deep Relaxation Practice: Cosmic Awareness ·
[15–30 minutes]

This deep relaxation practice is based on the practice known in Sanskrit as Shavaratra (Journey of the Corpse). It is the practice of animating the body with prana, which keeps the mind busy, withdraws your attention inward, and sharpens concentration as it moves from point to point in the body. It is traditionally taught by placing points of light in the body in a practice called *nyasa*, which means "to place" or "to plant." The widely taught practice places attention on points that are related to the marma points in the body. The origin of the practice can be traced to the Vasishtha Samhita and the Ayurvedic text, the Sushruta Samhita.[1] Other texts mention the importance of moving prana from point to point in the body as being the best practice of pratyahara.[2] I was first introduced to the practice of placing mantra in the body by Pandit Rajmani Tigunait during a teaching on Netra Tantra in 2005. I found it to be very powerful, so I offer a few suggestions below as options of what to place in the points.

You can follow the practice of placing points of light in the body, or you can customize the practice by choosing one of the following common options instead of light. Do not place fire or the sun in these points, and consult a qualified teacher before varying from this list.

AUM
The moon for soothing and nurturing
Your personal mantra (consult with your teacher)
Maha Mritjunjaya mantra for healing (page 187)
Rose-colored light for healing
The Sanskrit alphabet
A twinkling blue star (contraindicated for cancer or tumors)

Get into your yoga nidra nest and come to a comfortable resting position that you can stay in for 20 minutes with little to no movement. Of course, if you need to adjust during this time, permit yourself to do so.

Once you are settled in your resting position, allow your body to release even more by taking a few deep breaths. Feel your body resting on the earth. Notice your body breathing and feel its weight on the earth. Notice how your body gets lighter on the inhalation and heavier on the exhalation.

Feel the earth beneath you. Feel its strength, its solidity, and its unconditional support. Remember that the earth can hold the full weight of your body and anything else you may be carrying.

As you inhale, feel the earth rising up to hold you. As you exhale, feel the force of gravity and accept the invitation to release your full weight down, down, down into the earth. (2 minutes)

Become aware of the breath and notice where you feel it moving. Let the breath rise and fall in your belly (see Diaphragmatic Breathing, page 190).

With each breath in, feel how your body is refreshed and purified. With each breath out, feel yourself let go of all tension from both your body and your mind. (1 minute)

Begin to count the breaths backward from 20 to zero.

Inhale, 20; exhale, 20; inhale, 19; exhale, 19; and so on. Let go more and more until both your body and your mind feel free at zero. If you miss a number, start over again at 20. (2 minutes)

Let go of counting. Scan through your body to release any remaining tension. Remember your sankalpa:

May my mind be a flow of beautiful and divine
resolves, filled with auspicious thoughts. (1 minute)

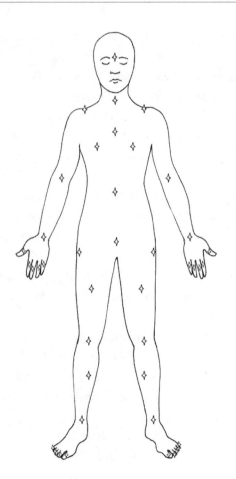

Bring awareness to the center point between your eyebrows; place a tiny star twinkling there. At each point that follows, see or place a twinkling star:

Pit of the throat
Right shoulder joint
Right elbow joint
Right wrist joint
Right pinky finger
Right ring finger
Right middle finger
Right index finger
Right thumb
Right wrist joint
Right elbow joint
Right shoulder joint
Pit of the throat
Left shoulder joint
Left elbow joint
Left wrist joint
Left pinky finger
Left ring finger
Left middle finger
Left index finger
Left thumb
Left wrist joint
Left elbow joint
Left shoulder joint
Pit of the throat
Center of the chest
Right nipple
   (or right side of the chest)

Left nipple
   (or left side of the chest)
Center of the chest
Navel center
Pelvic center
   (base of the spine)
Right hip joint
Middle of the right thigh
Right knee joint
Middle of the right calf
Right ankle joint
Right little toe
Right fourth toe
Right third toe
Right second toe
Right big toe
Right ankle joint
Middle of the right calf
Right knee joint
Middle of the right thigh
Right hip joint
Pelvic center
   (base of the spine)
Left hip joint
Middle of the left thigh
Left knee joint
Middle of the left calf
Left ankle joint

Left little toe	Pelvic center (base of the spine)
Left fourth toe	Navel center
Left third toe	Center of the chest
Left second toe	Right nipple
Left big toe	(or right side of the chest)
Left ankle joint	Left nipple
Middle of the left calf	(or left side of the chest)
Left knee joint	Center of the chest
Middle of the left thigh	Base of the throat
Left hip joint	Third eye center

See a constellation of stars in your body. See a constellation to the right and to the left of your body. Sense a galaxy of stars above your body. Sense a galaxy of stars below your body. Feel your whole body floating in a sea of starlight; your body is filled with this light. (3 minutes)

Let your awareness rest at your heart. Sense that your heart is filled with a sea of liquid diamonds. (10 minutes)

Rest in cosmic awareness. (3–10 minutes)

Remember that you have a body. Remember your sankalpa:

May my mind be a flow of beautiful and divine
resolves, filled with auspicious thoughts. (1 minute)

Now silently cognize where you are in space and time.
I am on planet Earth.
In the country of _____ .
In the state of _____ .
In the town of _____ .
In this room at _____ . (1 minute)
Deepen your breath. Begin to move your body in any way that feels intuitive,

such as doing long stretches or folding your knees into your chest. Welcome yourself back.

Roll to your right or left side. Notice how you feel. Take a few minutes to freewrite and then answer the self-inquiry questions.

SELF-INQUIRY

Directly after your deep relaxation practice, allow yourself 10 to 15 minutes to answer the following questions. Write as fast as you can. Don't worry about your grammar or sentence structure. Feel as though the flame at the altar of your heart is guiding your hand. You may answer the questions in words, poetry, dance, drawing, or painting. Just let it flow. As you continue with this practice, come back to these questions periodically and answer them again.

1. What are you asleep to in your life?
2. What price are you paying by remaining asleep?
3. What is the recurring pattern or theme in your life that remains in place by your choosing to stay asleep?
4. What is one thing that you can do every day to remind yourself to be present, compassionate, and courageous as you face life's challenges?
5. What is one thing that reinforces your tendency to stay asleep to the full potential of your life that you can *stop* doing every day?
6. What is one recurring thought that causes you discomfort in your life? Is it true? *How* does it keep you from moving forward?
7. What affirmation can you offer yourself that will keep you moving in a positive direction when you are feeling stuck?

DAILY PRACTICES

Choose at least one of the following shorter practices on days when you don't have time for deep relaxation and self-inquiry.

Bedtime Ritual: Mauna (Silence) *15 minutes*

Practice 15 minutes of silence before bedtime. Leave your phone in another room, turn off the TV, and unplug all the electronics in your bedroom so you can even eliminate the low hum and buzz of devices. Cover any electronics that might need to stay on with a towel or piece of dark material. If you are in a house with other people, make a plan with them to allow you to have some silence before bed. Notice the resistance that others may have to silence and have compassion. Use noise-canceling earphones, earplugs, a white noise machine, an Mp3 player, or an app. You may not have a full 15 minutes, but stay in silence as long as you can.

Let go of reading, texting, and planning. Just allow yourself to sit. Notice your breath, notice your body, notice your energy. Observe how your mind may want to have a conversation about what you are witnessing and let that go as well. Just come back to noticing, without needing to have a commentary or discussion with yourself about it. When you are ready to go to sleep, bring your awareness to your heart center and remember your sankalpa:

May my mind be a flow of beautiful and divine
resolves, filled with auspicious thoughts.

See the mantra as a light in your heart center or feel it as a vibration. Allow yourself to go to sleep as you hold this light or vibration in your heart.

Wake-Up Ritual: Mirror Gazing *5–10 minutes*

Sleep with a mirror by your bedside—an actual mirror, not the camera on your phone! Set your mental alarm clock (you can use your real alarm clock as a backup) for 15 minutes before you need to get out of bed. This way you will have time and space to practice.

As soon as you feel yourself waking up, remember that you are in the transition from sleeping to waking and savor the moment. Be present. After you have acknowledged the moment, reach for your mirror and look at yourself. Gaze into your own eyes. Do not look away. What do you see? Who do you see? What thoughts come to your mind about the reflection that is in front of you? What do you see in your eyes? Who are you?

Repeat out loud to yourself while gazing into your eyes: "I am worthy of the beauty of life." (3 times) Sit or get up, and freewrite for 3 minutes.

Nature-Amplification Practice: Starlight Activation *5 minutes*

Starlight Activation is one of my favorite nature practices to share on yoga nidra training retreats. Students feel so much more connected to the depths of yoga nidra by just doing this practice once. I intuitively practiced this in Big Sur one night on retreat and have been doing it ever since. It's perfect for when you are deep in nature with low light pollution, and you can see stars. Sometimes even in the city you can find a place where you can see the brightest star, Sirius, on a night with a new moon.

Find a safe place where you can lie down on a blanket or in a lounge chair, and gaze at the night sky. Keep your eyes open and your gaze soft. See the sky as a whole. Notice what you see. Now let your awareness move to a star that catches your attention. It might be one that is the brightest, is super blingy, or is part of your favorite constellation. Take a moment to remember that you are made of the same starlight.

Gaze at the star and then close your eyes. Continue to see the star and invite it to place itself in your body—right between your eyes at the third eye point. See it there, twinkling.

Now open your eyes again. See the star, close your eyes, and place the star in your midbrain. See it twinkling. Continue like this through your body. seeing the star and then placing it in your body. Don't worry if you don't see anything; feel the star, remember the star you just saw and imagine that you are placing it in your body.

Feel it twinkling in your throat, navel, and pelvic centers; at the base of your spine, at all your fingertips and toes. Fill your whole body with twinkling stars. See the galaxy inside you. Then open your eyes, see the sky above you filled with stars, close your eyes, and see the stars twinkling inside you. (5 minutes)

Feel yourself to be as expansive as the universe. Offer gratitude for the luminosity of the stars. If you aren't able to see the stars, try watching a video of starlight.[3]

Vritti Fire Offering

This is the practice of offering your thoughts—good, bad, or neutral—to the fire. Let it go!

Sit in front of a bonfire, fireplace, a candle, or any kind of open flame, or imagine yourself sitting in front of a roaring fire. Offer gratitude for the element of fire that purifies, transforms, and activates. Each time you have a thought, make a mental offering to the fire. We're not talking only of negative thoughts, but of positive and neutral thoughts too. Feel as though this fire has a cleansing quality to purify the lens through which you see and how you interpret the world.

For every thought that comes to your mind, make an offering. You can place your hand on your heart, reminding yourself that you are offering every single one of your thoughts from the heart with love and devotion.

Feel each offering into the fire making you feel lighter, less tense in body and mind. Feel all constriction and tension being actively subsumed by fire. Feel yourself becoming free in body and mind. Transformed. Clear. Renewed.

Take time to journal afterward, making notes of recurring thoughts and insights.

· 9 ·

Practice Four

The Light of Inner Knowing

THIS PRACTICE GUIDES you toward the cave of your heart, connecting you with your innermost flame (think, smallest Russian nesting doll). The supporting practices help to clear and create connection to the heart space and the light of inner knowing.

BENEFITS

Amplification of intuition
Connection to the light of inner knowing
Trust and self-reliance
Awakening to compassion and beauty

PRACTICE THIS . . .

- When you have deep questions or prayers that you hope to have answered.
- When you are ready to connect to deep knowing.

TEACH THIS . . .

- Only once you've practiced it and journaled about it daily for ninety consecutive days. This is an advanced practice. It's always essential to have an embodied experience, cultivated over time, of any practice before you share it with students.
- To experienced students who have been practicing with you and at home regularly and are ready to go deeper.

The practices in this chapter are for those times when you have a desire to develop a relationship with a part of you that is unchanging. Vedic wisdom tells us that there is a part of us that always knows and the practices in this chapter are dedicated to your inner knowing. In many traditions, the inner knowing is symbolized by a flame located in the heart: "The inextinguishable flame of awareness that follows us through every birth and death and through all our states of wakefulness, dreams, and deep sleep."[1] You can think of this flame as your inner teacher, wisdom, and knowing.

Our connection to our inner light allows us to move away from doubt, to let go of seeing others' opinions as more relevant or valuable than our own. It helps us take full responsibility for our own contentment and make choices that will allow us to thrive.

As I developed a relationship with my intuition, I began to notice that whenever I felt that sense of knowing, I also felt a distinct vibration or tingle in my body, like an electric current of truth. I began trying to tune in to this vibration deliberately, to lean into it, to trust it. I remembered other times in the past when I felt the same vibration very strongly, and it helped to alert me to things and people that were not in alignment with my truth, though many times it didn't make sense until much later. I also remembered those times I didn't pay attention to it and had to learn very hard lessons. When working with intuition, it's a great idea to write everything down so you have a record of what personal blind spots you uncover and how your intuition works.

I hope these practices will help you to build a relationship with your inner wisdom, enhance your ability to discern truth, and support you in cultivating the courage to listen deeply and act in ways that are in alignment with your truth.

PREPARING FOR DEEP RELAXATION

Moving the body, breath, and prana are great ways to prepare the body for rest. These preparatory practices are optional. When you can, take the time for them and notice how they support and enhance your experience.

Poses

Spend a few minutes in one or two of the following poses:

Gentle dynamic backbends linked to the breath—for example, poses such as Bhujangasana (Cobra Pose) and Salabhasana (Locust Pose)

Longer holds of heart-opening postures with HRIM—for example, Setu Bandha Sarvangasana (Supported Bridge Pose)

Pranayama

Take some time to explore this practice that is said to produce a relaxed state, calm anxiety and stress, and benefit the heart.[2] Take some time to journal afterward.

Bhramari Breath (Humming of the Bees, page 189) *3 minutes*

Prana Dharana (Vital Energy Concentration), ending with directing prana to the heart (page 191) *5 minutes*

Sankalpa

I connect with my inner light of knowing. In stillness and surrender, presence leads me to the truth, the eternal flame inside me that is the essence of knowledge and wisdom. In gratitude, I honor that eternal light.

Mantra

HRIM (*hreem*)

HRIM is a one-syllable sound related to the Goddess, the sun, and the heart, as well as *hridaya* (the spiritual heart center). It is said to activate the heart on all levels—physical, energetic, and spiritual.

· Deep Relaxation Practice: Altar of the Heart ·
[35 minutes]

Swami Lokeswarananda's translation of the ancient Sanskrit text the Chandogya Upanishad tells us that "within the body is an abode in the shape of a lotus [i.e., the heart], and within that there is a small space. One must search within this space and earnestly desire to know what is there."[3] The key to moving to a place of exploration is spaciousness and the ability to rest with a calm mind. Much can be revealed to us in the sacred space of the heart. This yoga nidra practice thrives with silence, patience, and stillness. Let go of looking for something to happen. Enter the practice with devotion and love for a part of yourself that you are ready to remember. This isn't a practice to rush. You'll need at least 45 to 60 minutes to do the practice and to process and digest the experience afterward. Try another practice in this chapter when you're short on time.

To prepare for the practice, spend a few minutes chanting AUM HRIM (*aum hreem*) with awareness at your heart center. (2 minutes)

Find a comfortable place to rest—in a chair, on the floor against the wall. Give yourself time to get comfortable in your nest. The most important thing is that you feel effortlessly supported. If you are sitting on a chair, feel the parts of your body that are touching the chair as being supported by the earth.

Bring your attention to the center of your chest, your spiritual heart. As your attention rests here, notice what you feel. Without judgment, just notice. Is there a lightness, a heaviness, constriction, space?

Feel acceptance arising as you observe whatever you find there and feel your body soften. As you breathe, what do you notice? Keeping your attention at your heart, feel as though you can breathe in and out from the heart space. As you exhale, breathe out with an audible, sweet sigh. Feel a sense of release and deepening relaxation with each breath. (9 breaths)

Now let your body settle into the floor. Make any last-minute adjustments for comfort. Feel the connection between your body and the earth. Notice each point of your body that connects to the earth. Feel yourself grounding into the earth through those points.

Begin to observe your breath. Notice the rise and fall of your navel center. As you inhale, feel your belly rise; as you exhale, feel it move toward your spine. Feel your breath becoming smoother and smoother, like a peaceful flow of breath in and out. Continue to watch your navel rise and fall. (2 minutes)

Feel as though you can relax each part of your body:

Forehead	Shoulders
Eyebrows	Chest
Eyes	Stomach
Nostrils	Navel
Cheeks	Pelvis
Jaw	Legs
Throat	Buttocks
Shoulders	Knees
Arms	Calves
Wrists	Feet
Hands	Toes
Fingers	

Feel your whole body relax, and observe the breath. Feel your whole body breathing. Begin to count your breaths backward from 20 to zero. Inhale, 20; exhale, 20; inhale, 19; exhale, 19; and so on. Each time you exhale, let go even more. Remember your sankalpa:

I connect with my inner light of knowing.
In stillness and surrender, presence leads me to the truth,
the eternal flame inside me that is the essence of knowledge
and wisdom. In gratitude, I honor that eternal light.

Feel your body breathing. Imagine you can draw the breath in through the top of your head. Feel the breath moving from the top of your head as you inhale and down and out of your navel as you exhale. (1 minute)

Inhale from the top of your head and exhale out of the heart center, the spiritual heart at the center of your chest. (1 minute)

Inhale from the top of your head and exhale out of the throat center. (1 minute)

Inhale from the top of your head and exhale out of the third eye. (1 minute)

Inhale from the top of your head and exhale through the throat center. (1 minute)

Inhale from the top of your head and exhale through the heart center. (1 minute)

Now feel the breath coming in through the heart center and going out through the heart center, as though the spiritual heart center itself was breathing. Feel the breath guiding you deeper into a place within you that is sacred. (1 minute)

Feel the breath guiding you deeper and deeper inside toward the cave of your heart. (2 minutes)

Each breath draws you deeper inside. (1 minute)

See a door to the innermost cave. (30 seconds) Push the door to the cave open. Inside the cave, you see an altar. (1 minute) Walk toward the altar, and take a comfortable seat in front of it. Notice all the items on the altar. There is a single candle flame there. See its color, its vibrancy. It is alive. (1 minute)

Take a few moments to connect with this flame—its light, its warmth, its knowing. (1 minute.) This flame is the part of you that knows and knows that it knows. (1 minute) Ask the flame any question that is in your heart. Listen carefully for the answer. Offer a prayer to the flame, and ask for anything you need in life. (2 minutes)

Now be here with the flame, keeping your awareness at your heart. Sit in front of the altar of your heart. Feel the walls of the cave expand with each out-breath and contract with each in-breath. (3 minutes)

The flame has a gift for you. Accept this gift and offer your gratitude to the flame. Offer gratitude to the part of yourself that is free from doubt and the stains of the mind. Remember that it is always within you.

Now just let go of doing and rest with all of your awareness deep in the cave of your heart. (3 minutes) Remember your sankalpa:

I connect with my inner light of knowing.
In stillness and surrender, presence leads me to the truth,
the eternal flame inside me that is the essence of knowledge
and wisdom. In gratitude, I honor that eternal light.

As you begin to awaken and deepen your breath, imagine this eternal light is guiding you. It will guide you to take your next breath, to move in a way that is supportive for you to come out of the practice, and to either come fully into the waking state or rest on your side. Listen to your inner knowing.

When you are ready to sit up, take a moment to welcome yourself back, and spend a few minutes freewriting about the answers to the questions you asked, the gift you received, and anything else you would like to remember.

SELF-INQUIRY

Directly after your deep relaxation practice, allow yourself 10 to 15 minutes to answer the following questions. Write as fast as you can. Don't worry about your grammar or sentence structure. Feel as though the flame at the altar of your heart is guiding your hand. You may answer the questions in words, poetry, dance, drawing, or painting. Just let it flow. As you continue with this practice, come back to these questions periodically and answer them again.

1. What is your relationship with intuition, or your inner knowing?
2. What does it feel like in your body?
3. What is your main obstacle to connecting with your inner knowing?
4. Do you let intuition guide your actions consistently? If not, why not?
5. Consider your relationship with intuition over the years. Has there ever been a time when you didn't listen to your

intuition, and there was a less-than-desirable result? When? What signs did you choose to ignore, and why?

6. When have you followed your intuition (maybe even against others' advice) and had it lead to a great outcome?
7. Take two minutes to write about the relationship between trust, courage, and intuition.

I recommend that people who wish to deepen their clarity and intuition commit to practicing Altar of the Heart for at least forty consecutive days. After this forty-day practice, answer the following questions:

- What is the biggest shift that has occurred in your life from doing a dedicated practice for forty days?
- What has been your most profound insight?

DAILY PRACTICES

Choose at least one of the following shorter practices on days when you don't have time for deep relaxation and self-inquiry.

Bedtime Ritual: Altar of Gratitude *5–15 minutes*

Before the practice, set your mental alarm clock for the time you would like to wake up in the morning. Lie down in Makarasana (Crocodile Pose, page 183). Fold your hands underneath your forehead, use the light pressure of your hands to draw the skin of the eyebrows down. Bring your awareness to your navel and feel it rising and falling.

Begin to practice 1:2 Breathing (page 191), inhaling for 3 seconds and exhaling for 6 seconds. Feel your rib cage expanding and your body relaxing. (6 minutes)

Before you go to sleep in whatever position you choose, bring your awareness to your heart and remember yourself sitting at the altar in front of the flame. See yourself placing an offering of gratitude into the flame. Allow awareness to stay at the heart center as you drift off to sleep.

If you find yourself waking up in the middle of the night, bring your attention back to your heart, offering gratitude to the flame. Let the flame be a constant presence as you move through the different stages of sleep.

Wake-Up Ritual: Connecting to Truth *5 minutes*

As you feel yourself begin to wake up, try not to jolt yourself awake. Feel into the space between sleep and wakefulness. Notice its liminal quality and savor it. Ask yourself, *What do I know to be true? If I follow this truth, where will it lead me?*

Spend a few minutes freewriting. If you don't have time to write, remember the answers to these questions and use them as a contemplation as you move through your day. Probe further by asking yourself, *Is this a thought that came from the mind? Or from the knowledge of the heart?*

This practice will help you tune in to feeling the difference between the frequencies of thinking and knowing.

Nature-Amplification Practice: Vast Blue Sky *3–10 minutes*

Find a quiet spot to lie down on the ground when the sky is clear and cloudless. If you live in a place that is perpetually cloudy, you can do this practice as a visualization, or just watch the sky as you get glimpses of blue. If it's not possible to lie down outside, you can also do this practice while standing or sitting, looking out of a window or using the power of imagination to remember a vast blue sky.

Place your hands on your belly and close your eyes. Notice your body breathing. Feel your belly rise and fall under the weight of your hands. Observe and smooth out any rough spots in your breath. Let your body soften a bit with each exhalation.

Open your eyes and gaze into the clear blue sky. The only movement in your body is your navel rising and falling. As you gaze into the sky, try to blink as little as possible. Continue to feel the rise and fall of your belly. (2 minutes)

As you continue to breathe, allow your chest to become more and more still as you breathe into your belly. Your navel is rising and falling. (1 minute)

Let your attention settle on the space of your heart. Feel your chest become more and more expansive. Imagine your entire chest becoming vast like the clear sky above you. Feel the sense of vastness spread to your belly, legs, arms, and head. Let vast expansiveness fill your whole body. (2 minutes)

Close your eyes and feel yourself as vast, expansive space. (5 minutes)

Come back to sitting, and spend 5 minutes freewriting.

Clearing the Heart Space Practice *3–10 minutes*

Lie on the earth or on the floor either in Savasana or on your back drawing the soles of your feet together and allowing your knees to splay out, adding support under your knees if needed. Prior to practice, you may want to let people know that you will be doing some loud exercises and not to disturb you.

Witness the breath. Notice the quality of mind; notice how they are linked. (1 minute) Let your awareness move to the space of your heart. Inhale with attention at the heart, and exhale with a sweet sigh. (9 breaths)

Be still and observe your breath. See a smoky gray thundercloud resting at your heart center. Take your biggest in-breath ever and hold it for a moment.

Visualize a big, bright, beautiful sun coming directly behind the cloud and beginning to dissolve it. Exhale with a scream of "Aahh" (as loud as you can!) as you see this cloud being dissolved by the bright sun. The cloud disperses as the rays of the sun begin to shine through.

Do this three to four more times, each time seeing the cloud dissolving more and more. Bang your hands on the ground and stomp your feet as you scream, and see this cloud completely disappear! The radiance of the sun is filling the heart space. Allow any emotions to release as the radiance fills the heart space.

Now be still. See and sense the beautiful radiance of the sun. Feel every part of your body active, alive, radiant, free, and joyful. Every cell of your body vibrating with radiance. (5 minutes)

When you feel complete, spend 5 minutes freewriting.

· 10 ·

Practice Five

Bliss Nectar Activation

THE LAST VERSE of the Ratri Suktum, which is included in this practice, is part of the prayer that Brahma sang to the Goddess Yoga Nidra to petition her help in waking Vishnu. It praises her moonlike and radiant beauty and nurturing qualities. It is the radiance of the moon that brings nurturing and healing nectar. These practices invoke all those qualities.

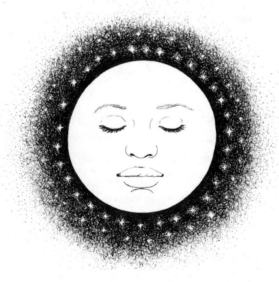

BENEFITS

Body/mind healing and nurturing
Calm mind
Contentment
Heart soothing

PRACTICE THIS . . .

- After a lot of activity, movement, or outward flowing energy. However, if your energy has been feeling dull or lethargic over a long period of time, try Practice Three in chapter 8 instead.
- On full moon and new moon nights.
- When you have ample time and won't be rushed.
- When you feel the need for nurturance and rejuvenation.

TEACH THIS . . .

- When you would like to invoke a powerful nurturing and healing tone for your class.
- To follow and balance a more dynamic asana practice.

Most of us put a lot of our energy out into the world on a daily basis. This practice invokes the qualities of the moon to refill your energetic cup and bring you back into balance. It heals and nurtures both the body and the mind by promoting contentment, soothing the heart, and calming the mind. To realize this overall healing effect, the practice should not be rushed but savored with a devotional quality acknowledging all is ready to be healed within you.

PREPARING FOR DEEP RELAXATION

Moving the body, breath, and prana are great ways to prepare the body for rest. These preparatory practices are optional. When you can, take the time for them and notice how they support and enhance your experience.

Poses

Spend a few minutes practicing one or two of the following:

> Moon Salutations (page 182)
> Salamba Sarvangasana (Supported Shoulderstand) with a peaceful
>   attitude (page 183)
> Dancing to your favorite music *5 minutes*

Pranayama

These are two of my favorite practices. Try Chandra Bhedana to bring forward a cooling, nurturing quality, and Circular Breathing to allow a sense of inner stillness to unfold. After practicing one of these pranayamas, take some time to freewrite in your journal about the effects.

Chandra Bhedana (Moon-Piercing Breath, page 189) *3 minutes*

Circular Breathing (page 189) *4 minutes*

Sankalpa

I receive the vibration of peace and bliss. I bathe in the vapors of the moon, allowing them to infuse every cell of my being with the healing nectar of infinite joy, purity, and divine nurturance.

Mantra

This mantra can be done anytime—even while you are washing the dishes.

SO HAM (*hum*)

I am that *5 minutes*

As you breathe in, you hear the mantra SO, and on the exhalation, you hear the mantra HAM as you feel waves of rejuvenation and prana expand through your body. This is not a practice of you repeating the mantra mentally. You are literally listening for the sound of the mantra as it rides on your inhalation (SO) and exhalation (HAM). SO HAM is the mantra we were all born with as it is the sound of the breath. It reminds us that we are all connected to something greater.

RATRI SUKTUM VERSE 10: Remember the story of Brahma singing praises to the Goddess Yoga Nidra to awaken Vishnu? This verse is part of that hymn. Take a moment to chant it under the moonlight when you feel a need for cooling and a calm, nurturing presence. *Saumya* means gentle in action; pearl-like; moonlike; evoking the qualities of purity, tranquility, and peacefulness.

> SAUMYĀ SAUMYĀTARĀŚEṢĀ
> SAUMYEBHYAS TVATI SUNDARI
> PARĀPARĀṆĀṀ PARAMĀ
> TVAMEVA PARAMESHVARĪ

> You are beauty and more beauty. You are most beautiful among all of the saumya things. You are Parameshwari, the Supreme Goddess beyond all the things near and far.

SRIM (*shreem*): SRIM relates to the moon; the goddess of prosperity, Lakshmi; and has a soothing effect on the mind. It is a perfect mantra to express our faith that we are held and supported by forces seen and unseen. SRIM also relates to our blissful and radiant nature to shine.

· Deep Relaxation Practice: Healing Moon Nectar ·
[25–40 minutes]

Find a comfortable and safe place to practice. Decide how you will set yourself up—lying down, lying on your side, or sitting against a wall. Create your yoga nidra nest and come to your resting position. Begin by feeling your body resting on the ground. Notice your body breathing. Feel the earth beneath you. (2 minutes)

Imagine drawing a circle of protection around your body, then another circle around that, and one more larger circle around that. See and feel yourself lying inside the inner circle. (1 minute)

Listen for the most distant sounds that you can hear. Letting go of judgment or the need to analyze, let your attention move from sound to sound to sound. Imagine the sounds in your environment are outside the circles. Just let them be there. (2 minutes)

Observe your body breathing. Feel the earth beneath you as you watch your navel rise and fall. (2 minutes)

As you inhale, feel the earth rising up to hold you. As you exhale, allow your body to release into the earth. Feel the support of the earth. Let the earth receive your body. (2 minutes)

Feel your body breathing and imagine you could direct the breath in through your left nostril and exhale out of the right. You are just using the power of the mind; where your mind goes, your energy goes. (2 minutes) Now switch. Inhale through your right nostril, and exhale through the left. (2 minutes)

Now begin to count the breath backward from 18 with every exhalation. Inhale right, 18; exhale left, 18; inhale left, 17; exhale right, 17; and so on. As you exhale, feel your body and mind release deeper layers of tension. Keep going until you get to zero. If you miss a number, start back at 18. (2 minutes)

Let go of counting and experience the essence of being. (1 minute) Remember your sankalpa:

> I receive the vibration of peace and bliss. I bathe in the vapors
> of the moon, allowing them to infuse every cell of my being with
> the healing nectar of infinite joy, purity, and divine nurturance.

Notice the flow of the breath and feel it moving in your spine. See a full moon at the base of your spine. As you breathe in, feel the moon travel up your spine to the crown of your head. As you exhale, the moon sends nurturing energy down into your entire body. (9 breaths)

Bring your awareness to the third eye, the point between your eyebrows on the surface of your skin. Sense a drop of luminous healing nectar there. It's as if the moon had flowers; this is the nectar from those flowers. Hear the healing mantra SRIM, the mantra of radiance, love, and prosperity. Bring awareness to points in your body. Feel, sense, or see a drop of healing nectar at each point and hear the mantra SRIM:

Third eye SRIM
Right eye SRIM, healing nectar
Left eye SRIM, healing nectar
Right ear
Left ear
Right nostril
Left nostril
Right cheek
Left cheek
Upper lip
Lower lip
Upper teeth
Lower teeth
Throat center SRIM
Right shoulder

Right elbow
Right wrist
Right thumb
Right index finger
Right middle finger
Right ring finger
Right pinky finger
Right wrist
Right elbow
Right shoulder
Throat center
Left shoulder
Left elbow
Left wrist
Left thumb

Left index finger
Left middle finger
Left ring finger
Left pinky finger
Left wrist
Left elbow
Left shoulder
Throat center
Heart center
Left side of the chest
Right side of the chest
Navel
Pelvic center
Base of spine
Right hip
Right knee
Right ankle
Right big toe
Right second toe
Right third toe
Right fourth toe
Right pinky toe

Right ankle
Right knee
Right hip
Pelvic center
Left hip
Left knee
Left ankle
Left big toe
Left second toe
Left third toe
Left fourth toe
Left pinky toe
Left ankle
Left knee
Left hip
Pelvic center
Navel center
Heart center
Right side of the chest
Left side of the chest
Throat center
Third eye

Feel that your entire body is filled with the cooling, immortal nectar of the moon. Your whole body is vibrating with the frequency and vibration of SRIM. Sense your whole body being filled with nectar. Feel yourself floating in a cloud of moonlight—healing, nurturing, rejuvenating. Feel the vibration of SRIM throughout your body. (2 minutes)

Bring your awareness to the throat center, and see a full moon at your throat. (2 minutes)

Let your awareness rest at your heart center. (7 minutes)
Remember your sankalpa:

I receive the vibration of peace and bliss. I bathe in the vapors
of the moon, allowing them to infuse every cell of my being with
the healing nectar of infinite joy, purity, and divine nurturance.

Slowly begin to deepen your breath. Remember where you are. Remember
that you have a body. Notice how you feel.

Turn onto your side and practice side lying for a few breaths. When you
feel ready, come up to a seated posture. Spend 3 minutes freewriting.

SELF-INQUIRY

Directly after your deep relaxation practice, allow yourself 10 to 15 minutes to
answer the following questions. Write as fast as you can. Don't worry about
your grammar or sentence structure. Feel as though the flame at the altar
of your heart is guiding your hand. You may answer the questions in words,
poetry, dance, drawing, or painting. Just let it flow. As you continue with this
practice, come back to these questions periodically and answer them again.

1. In what environments do you feel most at ease?
2. With whom do (did) you feel most at ease? With whom can
   you be your most authentic self?
3. How easily can you move past anger? What are your tools?
4. Which activities bring you the most joy?
5. Describe a time in your past when you felt blissful. Give details:

   What were you doing?
   What season was it?
   Where were you?

6. How can you cultivate more time for joyful experiences and heart-centered friendships in your life?

DAILY PRACTICES

Choose at least one of the following shorter practices on days when you don't have time for deep relaxation and self-inquiry.

Bedtime Ritual: Moon Dream *5 minutes*

The center of the dreaming state is located at the throat center and symbolized by a full moon. Prepare yourself for bed with anywhere from 5 to 30 minutes of silence, if possible. If it is not feasible for you to be silent, softly hum the mantra AUM SRIM between conversations with loved ones and remember the qualities of the moon as you hum. Feel the mantra redirecting your awareness inward.

Remember to set your mental alarm clock for the time you want to get up the next morning. If it is a full moon night and you can see the moon: Gaze at the moon and feel as though you can inhale the vapors of the moon as if you are sipping through a giant straw.

When you are in bed, lie on your back and close your eyes. Visualize a full moon resting at the throat center. With your attention on that moon, repeat the sankalpa three times:

I receive the vibration of peace and bliss. I bathe in the vapors of the moon, allowing them to infuse every cell of my being with the healing nectar of infinite joy, purity, and divine nurturance.

Let yourself drift off to sleep.

Wake-Up Ritual: Soma Beauty Ritual *3 minutes*

As you feel yourself beginning to emerge from sleep, linger in the pause and remember that this transition is an extremely potent space to create a theme for your day.

In that space of transition, remember the moon at your throat and allow it to rise into your face. Relax your face, relax your forehead, and release any tension in your jaw. Feel the flow of your breath.

Repeat to yourself, *I embody bliss. Bliss is my true nature.* Feel the corners of your mouth turn upward. Repeat again, *I embody bliss. Bliss is my true nature.*

Continue this contemplation throughout the day. It is said that one who has a moonlike face is a sought-after friend.

Nature-Amplification Practice:
Saumya Activation *5–10 minutes*

Practice this under a full moon. If you are somewhere where you cannot see the moon, try this: On a full moon night, find a color photo of the full bright moon against a black background from the NASA online library. Sit three to four feet away from your computer and turn off all the lights.

Sit in a comfortable position in a chair, on the ground in meditation pose, or leaning against a wall or tree. Gaze at the moon and take a few moments to contemplate the quality of the quality of the moonlight—cooling, nurturing, and peaceful. Offer your gratitude for all these qualities and remember what they feel like in your body.

Practice Chandra Bhedana (Moon-Piercing Breath, page 189). Imagine a tiny version of the moon hanging near your left nostril. Imagine inhaling the vapors of the moon through your left nostril and exhaling out of the right.

Inhale and silently repeat AUM.

Exhale and silently repeat SRIM.

As you inhale and exhale, sense that your body is being restored and rejuvenated. (10 breaths)

Now lie down and feel yourself bathing in moonlight as you gaze at the moon. Feel the moonlight rising through both nostrils. As you close your eyes, imagine you are inhaling moonlight as breath into your body. (1 minute)

See a full moon at your throat center. (1 minute) See it rising into your face as a full, bright moon. Sense and feel your entire face is a radiant full moon. (1 minute)

Feel moonlight begin to fill your whole body. With each breath, your body fills with the healing nectar and frequency of the moon. (1 minute)

Feel moonlight spreading beyond the physical confines of your body and filling the space around you. Feel yourself cocooned in moonlight. (2 minutes)

Feel that you are the moon—peaceful, silent, nurturing, and whole.

SING TO THE MOON. LEARN THE LAST VERSE OF THE RATRI SUKTUM. For an entire moon cycle of thirty days, go outside, look for the moon, and sing the last verse of the hymn to it. Remember her phase from the night before. If you cannot see the moon, just remember how she looked the last time you saw her and sing. Sing with gratitude for her beauty, radiance, and qualities of embracing change with grace and steadiness. This is a great practice for teachers of yoga nidra to incorporate as part of daily practice.

Take a few minutes after each session to draw the phase of the moon in your journal and freewrite for 2 minutes. If you are in a place where you cannot see the moon, start on a full moon night. Visualize the moon and her phases, sing, and practice journaling each night for thirty days.

· 11 ·

Practice Six
Into the Void

THIS PRACTICE IS a journey beyond the elemental world. It moves you toward greater expansion and cosmic awareness.

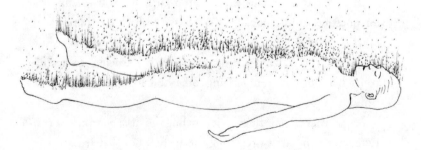

BENEFITS

Clarity
Creativity
Inspiration
Transformation
Oneness

PRACTICE THIS . . .

- To activate your creativity and inspiration.
- After spending a few months consistently working with the deep relaxation and nature-amplification practices in the earlier chapters. It is essential to build the discipline to remain present to the part of you that can stay awake and aware while in practice, even though the physical body may be sleeping.

TEACH THIS . . .

- Only once you have dedicated yourself to consistent practice. Use your sharpened discernment to decide if and when to share this practice. Try it one-on-one with a fellow teacher or longtime student who also has a committed practice. This practice should not be shared in groups that are too large for you to support for questions and feedback. Before you embark on sharing the practice, you must give yourself an attitude adjustment—shift your perspective from seeing yourself as a teacher to seeing yourself as one who is practicing something in order to learn and embody it.
- When you have ample time for journaling and discussion afterward. Remember, the art of teaching the techniques that lead to the

grace of yoga nidra is sacred. Your students may have profound experiences that they need time to process afterward.

If you have made it this far, I imagine you have a deep desire to know another part of yourself that you may have glimpsed in other practices or maybe just by watching a beautiful sunrise. You know that you are more than your body, and you may feel that there is more to reality than what you see with your two eyes. This practice can offer you a peek through the doorway into another dimension of reality. It may change you.

It is essential to build the discipline to remain present to the part of you that can stay awake and aware while in practice, even though the physical body may be sleeping.

This is not to say that the grace of Nidra Shakti is linear in any way, because it isn't. All of the deep relaxation and nature-amplification practices you have done so far have been mere preparation. It is all we can do—make ourselves ready. The more we practice relaxing deeply while staying awake and aware, the more we can let go of expectation, of trying to have an "experience" or see something sublime. The fact is that the sublime is already present. We just don't know where to look. Yoga nidra guides us inward where all the treasures are found.

As you enter this practice, do so with reverence and devotion for the essence of yoga nidra. Recall the experiences you have had so far. Imagine gathering up all the healing, inspiration, aha moments, and fruits of your practice like flowers in a basket. Take a moment to center yourself and make an offering of your basket of flowers to the altar of your own heart, the Goddess, or your ancestors as you prepare to enter this practice.

PREPARING FOR YOGA NIDRA PRACTICE

Moving the body, breath, and prana are great ways to prepare the body for rest. These preparatory practices are optional. When you can, take the time for them and notice how they support and enhance the experience.

Poses

Spend a few minutes practicing one of the following poses while remaining aware of your breath:

Savasana (Corpse Pose, page 183)
Makarasana (Crocodile Pose, page 183)

Pranayama

Choose any one of the following to practice, notice its effects, and make notes.

1:2 Breathing (page 191) *10 minutes*

Nadi Shodhana (Alternate Nostril Breathing, page 190) *10–15 minutes*

Diaphragmatic Breathing (page 190) *10 minutes*

Shusumna Meditation (page 192) *5 minutes*

Sankalpa

I am as vast as the dark night sky, both empty and full. I surrender to grace. I am awake to the infinite space of the eternal; my creativity, inspiration, and potential are boundless.

Mantra

Sit in your meditation posture, bring your attention to the base of your spine and your connection to the earth. Mentally or verbally chant the mantras.

KRIM (*kreem*), AUM (*aum*) *5 minutes*

KRIM is the seed mantra of the goddess Kali, who rules over time, space, and action. AUM is the sound of creation and the higher self.

· Yoga Nidra Practice ·
[50 minutes]

By now, you have created your perfect yoga nidra nest. Remember to tend to parts of your body that need more support, padding, or warmth. You are preparing to let the body go, to let the mind and thoughts dissolve, and to allow yourself to receive the grace of the Goddess Yoga Nidra. Spare no luxury for yourself in your setup. This is not a time to skimp!

Prior to practice, remember the sankalpa:

I am as vast as the dark night sky, both empty and full.
I surrender to grace. I am awake to the infinite space of the eternal; my creativity, inspiration, and potential are boundless.

Begin the practice in Makarasana (Crocodile Pose, page 183) to prepare. Feel your hands on your forehead drawing your eyebrows down. Begin Diaphragmatic Breathing (page 190). Feel your navel rise and fall and your rib cage inflate as you breathe in and out. Slowly find a 1:2 breath ratio, inhaling for a count of 3 and exhaling for 6.

If your breath capacity can handle more volume, you can increase the inhalation and then double the length of the exhalation. You should not be straining—iron out any sounds or breaks in your breath. Make the breath as smooth and tranquil as possible. Feel your navel rising and falling. (3 minutes)

Roll over to your right side and feel the breath entering your left nostril. Imagine the whole left side of your body is breathing. Feel a sense of coolness and nurturing entering your body. (1 minute)

Roll over to your left side in the fetal position and breathe through your right nostril. Feeling as though the entire right side of your body is breathing. (1 minute)

Now turn and position yourself for deep relaxation. Take a moment to make an offering or prayer from your heart to the Goddess Yoga Nidra, your inner teacher, a beloved teacher, or guide. Draw a circle of protective light around you if desired.

Begin to breathe through both nostrils equally. See or sense the flow of breath moving through the central channel of your spine. As you inhale, silently repeat AH; as you exhale, repeat HAM (*hum*). (1 minute)

Now let go of the mantra and notice the sounds in the space around you. Let your awareness jump from sound to sound to sound, letting go of judgment about them. (1 minute) Let all the sounds be there. You are inside your protected circle, and all the sounds are on its circumference. (2 minutes)

Feel the earth beneath you and notice your body breathing. Feel prana riding on the breath as you breathe. Bring awareness to your spine. Silently chant AH as you inhale, feeling the sound rise from the base of your spine to the crown, and HAM as you exhale, feeling the sound descend down from the crown of your head to the base of your spine. (2 minutes)

Feel all the points of your body that are connected to the floor, and feel your body relax.

Feel where your heels connect to the earth.

Notice which parts of your legs connect to the earth.

Feel where your buttocks and the ground connect.

Notice the parts of your spine that connect to the earth.

Feel the contact point between your shoulder blades and the earth.

Feel the back of your head and where it connects to the earth.

Feel all the parts of your body that are connected to the earth.

Feel each exhalation grounding you and relaxing your body more and more.

Feel all the parts of your body that are connected to the earth. (1 minute)

Feel the space between your body and the earth. Feel all the parts of your body that are not connected to the earth. (1 minute) Feel breath and prana moving up and down your spine. Silently repeat AH as you inhale and HAM as you exhale. Each time you exhale HAM, feel your body release a little more. (9 breaths)

Bring your awareness to your toes. Feel the presence of prana. Inhale and feel a wave of prana traveling from the tips of your toes all the way to the crown of your head. As you exhale, the wave of prana moves back down to the soles of your feet. (4 minutes)

With your next breath, feel the wave from your ankles to the top of your head and back down to your ankles. (4 minutes)

Feel prana move from your knees to the top of your head and back to your knees. (3 minutes)

Follow prana from your hips to the crown of your head and back to your hips as you exhale. (2 minutes)

Watch prana and presence move from your navel center to the crown of your head and back to your navel as you exhale. (2 minutes)

Observe the wave from the heart center to the crown of your head and back to the heart center as you exhale. (2 minutes)

Watch prana move from the throat center to the crown of your head and back to the throat center as you exhale. (2 minutes)

Inhale and sense the wave move from your third eye to the crown of your head and back to your third eye point as you exhale. (3 minutes)

Inhale and sense presence move from the guru chakra (the point between the third eye and crown) to the crown of your head and back to the guru chakra as you exhale. (5–7 minutes)

Let your awareness settle at the third eye. Feel the breath moving in and out from this point. (1 minute) Move your awareness to the throat center and feel presence moving in and out. (1 minute) Move your awareness to the heart center and feel presence moving in and out. (3 minutes)

Still resting awareness at your heart, imagine the space below your body as a dark void, inky black space. Feel the space above your body as a dark void. (1 minute) The space to the right of your body is a dark void, and to the left of your body is dark space. (1 minute)

The space above your head is a void, dark space.

Below your feet is a void, dark, black space.

Sense the space inside your body as a void, dark space.

Feel that you are presence floating in the void. You are empty dark space.

Rest in and as the void. (10 minutes)

Rest in spaciousness.

Bring awareness back to the heart center. Feel the breath moving in and out from the heart center. Repeat AH as you inhale and HUM as you exhale. (9 times)

Let awareness rest at each of the energy centers in your body:

Third eye—breathe in and out.
Throat center—breathe in and out.
Heart center—breathe in and out.
Navel center—breathe in and out.
Pelvic center—breathe in and out.
Base of the spine—breathe in and out.

Slowly welcome yourself back. Take your time. Deepen your breath. Slowly move your fingers. Savor the liminal space for moment. Gently rise up to sitting.

SELF-INQUIRY

Directly after your yoga nidra practice, allow yourself 10 to 15 minutes to answer the following questions. Write as fast as you can. Don't worry about your grammar or sentence structure. Feel as though the flame at the altar of your heart is guiding your hand. You may answer the questions in words, poetry, dance, drawing, or painting. Just let it flow. As you continue with this practice, come back to these questions periodically and answer them again.

1. What was your experience of sensing your body suspended in space without support?
2. What emotions or thoughts did you feel arising?
3. Describe what emerged for you in this practice. What did you see, feel, or hear?

4. Was there anything about this experience that felt familiar? If so, describe how in detail.

DAILY PRACTICES

Choose at least one of the following shorter practices on days when you don't have time for yoga nidra and self-inquiry.

Bedtime Ritual: I AM *5–10 minutes*

Set your mental alarm clock for the morning and go to sleep with your attention at the heart center. Close your eyes, and just notice the darkness. Begin to notice your breath. Let go of judging and just notice.

Notice the aromas in the air. (1 minute) Notice the feeling of the sheets on your skin and which parts of your body are touching the bed. (1 minute) Notice any taste in your mouth.

Listen to your breath and notice all the sounds around you. Notice the sounds of your breath, your heartbeat, the fluids moving in your body. (2 minutes)

Feel your awareness becoming more internal as you let go. Allow presence to guide you deeper within. Follow that presence to the center of your chest— your spiritual heart center.

Remember the mantra (this is one of the "great utterances" known as Mahavakya):[1]

AHAM BRAHMAMSI

I am the Absolute.

With that mantra on your heart, drift off to sleep.

Wake-Up Ritual: I Am Awake *3 minutes*

As you feel yourself waking up, remember the void. Every transition holds a little yoga nidra: the space between the in-breath and the out-breath; the moments between twilight and sunrise, the sun setting and the rise of the moon, the blinking of your eyes. Notice the transitions (your breath, light filtering into your eyes, distant sounds) that are occurring just in the first few moments of waking.

Repeat to yourself, *I am awake to the infinite space of the eternal; my creativity, inspiration, and potential are boundless. The transitions are portals to expanded awareness and magic. I am awake to my life.*

Remember that there is a part of you that stays awake through all the states of consciousness. It is this part of yourself that you come to know during the practice of yoga nidra. Continue this contemplation throughout the day.

Lessons from the Void *10–20 minutes*

Take a moment to find a place where you can be in the dark—pitch-black darkness. I like to do this practice in the middle of the forest or nature, but if that is not convenient for you, you can do it in a dark room. Practice somewhere you feel safe and won't be disturbed. Let others know that you are doing a practice for 10 to 20 minutes.

Sit in your comfortable seat with your eyes slightly open. Gaze into the darkness in front of you. (3 minutes) Ask yourself, *How can I partner with the unknown? What is my greatest fear? What tools can help me to transform fear? Whom can I share my fears with in a safe space?* Notice what feelings arise within you.

You are not trying to see anything except the dark void in front of you. Feel yourself sinking into the void. Withdraw your senses inward. Feel your attention expanding into the infinite space of the void.

If you feel afraid of the dark or have experienced trauma, please consult with a therapist or practice this with a trusted friend before embarking on it alone. Take several minutes to freewrite about this practice. What did you learn? What information have you gained that can help you hold both fear and courage simultaneously?

Conclusion

The True Secret to Freedom

Deep relaxation and yoga nidra are profound practices for exploring your relationship with yourself, the world around you, and the Divine. Yoga nidra is a full system of yoga that can lead to the highest states of spiritual freedom (*moksha*).

How do you get there? How will you know when you do? The American founder of Viniyoga, Gary Kraftsow, has answered these questions. He says moksha is "achieved not by knowing the truth but awakening to it as a lived experience. Do the practice until it becomes a lived experience, and then you will know."[1]

You cannot think your way to spiritual freedom. It is not a gift of the intellect. It is an embodied experience that comes with consistent practice and grace. Once you possess this knowledge, no one can ever take it away from you. It becomes the foundation that supports your life and buoys up all your other practices and endeavors. This is a result of dedicated sadhana (committed practice or means of accomplishing something).

CHANGE YOUR BRAIN

A consistent practice, performed over a long period of time and with devotion, will change you. Consistency can help you to create new habits, open up new levels of understanding, and activate a new level of discipline and willpower.

Imagine activating a new self that is programmed for freedom. With practice, you can. Joe Dispenza, a neuroscientist and author of *Evolve Your*

Brain, explains that each time you make a choice that is aligned with your goal of spiritual freedom (for example, trying any of the practices, no matter how short), "you are priming your brain to install the neurological hardware to actually think, act, and feel like the person you want to be in your future. If you keep firing and wiring those networks in your brain, the hardware eventually becomes the software program, and making choices that are in alignment with your future becomes more automatic. When you do it enough times, as we walk as our future self—as we get our body involved each day in the process—this behavior becomes the habit of the new self."[2]

This is the wisdom behind doing a practice over an extended period. All the efforts you make to be consistent with your practice—whether it is for three minutes or an hour a day—will pay off with more stability and clarity.

TAPAS AND CHANGE

This is where a thirty- to ninety-day sadhana comes in. Sadhana creates *tapas*, translated as "heat"; "discipline"; or practices that lead to a clarity of the body, mind, and senses. The heat of tapas arises from the friction caused by our practice going against the grain of our habits and preferences. For example, tapas, in deep relaxation, may involve you committing to staying awake and aware during the practice as opposed to falling asleep. Committing to doing something every day, no matter what, is a powerful form of tapas for most of us. It means you can't miss a day or risk having to start over from day one. Keep in mind that your sadhana doesn't have to be all that long to be effective: start with mini-sadhanas lasting three to five consecutive days to get warmed up. This builds your inspiration to devote yourself to longer practices. I like to think that the longer the sadhana lasts, the more radiance and growth can come from it. So why not make life a radiance sadhana? Weaving the Householder's Flow into your practice can soften the masculine edges of discipline and transform discipline into devotion. Have compassion for yourself, and keep the thread of sadhana alive even when you can't do a long practice each day.

Under stay-at-home orders during the COVID-19 pandemic, we were all forced into a global sadhana of sorts—months of changing our habits, surrendering our preferences, and getting still. As a collective, we all endured something that we previously might have thought was intolerable. Many people faced the discomfort, adapted, and became stronger as a result. Still, we collectively suffered great losses from which we could not look away. The global stillness led to many things that we were previously too distracted to see or acknowledge and allowed them to come into clear and undeniable focus. We have the capacity to gain more clarity and self-knowledge if we stay awake to the lessons and don't run from the heat or friction produced in the discomfort. This is the alchemy of spiritual transformation.

Imagine that the very resistance we have toward staying consistent, committed, and awake in practice can help us to activate creativity, clarity, and inner radiance. It requires us to pull together all the energy that usually flows outward toward distraction and the external and use it as a sacred offering for our practice, healing, and transformation. Anything that we genuinely want to manifest requires effort and clarity of intention. This is how our devotion to practice will help us long after the sadhana is over. Shivani—a mother of twins, lawyer, and wife who attended a yoga teacher training with me—shared these thoughts at the end of a thirty-day commitment to practice:

> At the end of the thirty days, I felt an internal stillness and quiet. It was a sense of confidence or faith in self that I've never known before . . . a state of being. It was contentment beyond the everyday stresses and realities of being a working mother with young children. Yoga nidra even shifted things in a positive way in my relationships with others—my husband and my children. I was softer, more patient, more loving. I felt I had access to greater internal resources during times of stress. I am still in awe of the power of this one practice to transform from the inside out.

AWARENESS AT THE HEART:
THE PORTAL TO TRUTH

Chapter 2 described the sacred portals, but it's worth highlighting the heart center again as a place to explore. Verse 15 of the Shiva Sutras, as translated by Pandit Rajmani Tigunait, reads "by focusing the mind at the heart, a yogi gains knowledge of what is part of the waking and dreaming states."[3] Awareness at the heart connects you to the part of yourself that knows and is also the energy center associated with deep sleep. Practicing rituals mentally in the heart center is one of the most profound forms of pratyahara, which you may remember from earlier chapters as being one of the limbs of yoga and central to deepening your relaxation and yoga nidra practices. By now you have hopefully tried many of the practices in this book and noticed that, at the end of them, you are often asked to rest awareness at the heart. This is all in preparation for entering the space at the heart center and receiving the grace of yoga nidra. Practice leading yourself through the simplest of relaxations and then let awareness rest at your heart center for between 3 and 10 minutes. This is where you reap the benefits of your devotion to a consistent practice and discover just how simple the practice can be. The heart center is where the human and the Divine meet. During the practice, you may begin to notice that you feel a certain frequency or vibration that carries a nurturing tone. With consistency, this becomes an inner vibration or fragrance that stays with you long after your practice is completed. Tune in to this vibration and learn to recognize it; this vibration holds wisdom and healing.

SELF-INQUIRY

When we practice deep relaxation, it is devotion, deep surrender, and the fruit of all the other practices that came before that can lead us to the grace of yoga nidra. How we enter the practice, our intentions for practicing, what we think as we lie down to practice can all influence the experience.

Pause and take a few moments to answer the following questions to help you clarify the deeper aspects of your practice.

1. What does your heart long for in relation to your spiritual practice?
2. How do you connect to devotion in your practices?
3. How has your concept or understanding of surrender evolved since beginning the practices of deep relaxation?
4. What is your biggest fear about letting go?
5. What distractions are you ready to release to empower your practices?
6. Is there any resistance to practice that seems insurmountable?
7. List three things that may be an antidote to this resistance.
8. What does it mean to be free? Is it possible to be free if others in this world are not free also?

SELF-GUIDING YOUR YOGA NIDRA PRACTICE

This may be the biggest secret the "yoga industry" doesn't want me to tell you: my practice began to take on new dimensions when I stopped listening to recordings and started guiding my practice myself. It turns out that *you* are the secret. If you are interested in deepening your experiences, I wholeheartedly encourage you to start a forty-day practice in which you lead yourself through deep relaxation, rest in deep surrender, and then follow prana back to its source. Let your attention rest at one of the sacred portals—the third eye, the throat, the womb, or the heart center. It could be so simple if only it weren't for resistance! Notice what comes up when you consider the idea of *guiding yourself* through the practice.

Doing a self-led practice gave me new insight into types of resistance that were not apparent when I was listening to a recording. I got a more in-depth look at my beliefs and my feelings about worthiness, safety, and even my physical body structure just from switching to self-guided practices. This is why I'm making a case for you to explore it as part of your sadhana if you want to experience the depths of what this practice can offer.

If yoga nidra is indeed the practice of remaining awake and aware through all the transitions of waking, dreaming, and deep sleep, then we need to learn how to be truly awake. If turiya (the fourth state) is also the state of *nirvikalpa* (no thought), it follows that having a recording playing during practice may at some point limit how much we can transcend. That's not to say you cannot have profound experiences using a recording because you absolutely can and do, but if you want to embrace the exploration of what it means to be free and embrace your power, I suggest to start experimenting with self-guided practices. Besides, it's said that the teachings were "revealed" to the rishis and rishikas. I imagine them deep in nature, observing the movement of the stars, moon, sun, and animals in silence and being guided by intuition and prana.

Some of the hidden practices of yoga nidra involve merging your consciousness with that of another being, generally one that is no longer on this earthly plane. Some say that is how lineage holders continue to receive teachings long after their gurus have died. Yet I have heard of students who have connected with the energy of loved ones who have passed over without any initiation into a particular practice. This practice holds power that we may never fully know in one lifetime.

Yoga nidra can be both a teacher and a path to higher awareness if you cultivate the ability to listen deeply and surrender to its grace. Once you begin self-guiding your practices, you will develop a profoundly personal relationship with the many aspects of yoga nidra, and that is where the real magic begins.

As part of the Empowered Wisdom Yoga Nidra training that I co-lead with Chanti Tacoronte-Perez, we ask students to do a forty-day self-practice as part of their ten-month journey toward teacher certification. We are usually met with looks of disbelief—"How in the world do you lead yourself through deep relaxation?"

There are a few steps that will help you begin to self-guide. Committed and devoted practice is the water that allows the wisdom of an embodied practice to blossom. This wisdom is a foundation that will support you the whole of your life. This type of wisdom cannot be lost or stolen. It is the kind of wisdom that will make us a good future ancestor. Remember though, wisdom can be forgotten, and this is why freewriting after practice is so important.

Ideas for Practicing Self-Guiding

- Do at least two forty-day sadhanas of one of the deep relaxation practices; use the same recording for all forty days. Choose the practice that you would like to self-guide and begin to commit it to memory. (Tips: Make a handwritten copy of the practice from the book. Transcribe the practice from the recording. Set an intention to memorize the practice while you are doing it.)
- Train yourself to wake up with your mental alarm clock (page 42).
- Practice either the 108 Countdown (page 193) or the Dream Stone practice (page 192).
- Keep both a yoga nidra practice journal and a dream journal: journal, freewrite, draw, or write poetry. Keeping a journal for your dreams can be helpful because they may become more lucid as you begin to self-guide your yoga nidra practices.
- Begin with a straightforward practice of relaxing your body parts and allowing your body to surrender, feeling all the places where the body and mind are holding on. You can do this practice upon waking, prior to sleeping, even when you are washing the dishes or talking on the phone with your ex. Perform this practice consistently for a minimum of one week.
- Do the wake-up and bedtime rituals as bookends to your day.
- Get outside and be in nature. Do some of the nature-amplification practices.

- Practice 30 minutes of silence either upon waking or before going to bed. No texting, listening to music, reading, or meditation. Just enjoy silence. Notice how your mind will want to begin a conversation. When this happens, take three deep breaths and return to silence.

Ten Steps to Self-Guiding Your Practice

When you are ready to try self-guiding, choose one of the practices from the preceding section and follow these steps:

1. Begin to lead yourself through your chosen practice.
2. Set an intention that you will remain awake and aware through the practice. If you feel yourself drifting off, remind yourself, "I am awake and aware." It's okay if you feel your physical body falling asleep and your mind letting go; consciousness remains awake.
3. Let go of feeling like you need to memorize something in order to "get it right." You are "memorizing" in order to know the steps; soften the edges around using the same exact words and phrases. Feel into it and guide yourself. Learn the foundations and origins of practice, explore some of the endnotes, then let your embodied experience and recollection of the practice guide you. Trust yourself and make notes about your experience. Share notes with other friends or teachers interested in yoga nidra.
4. To start, you can silently speak to yourself as though you are guiding another person. Imagine seeing yourself lying down as your own student and begin to guide yourself through the steps. Instead of saying, "Relax my right leg," change it to "Right leg relax." This will help you begin to create some distance between you and your body.
5. Observe yourself following your own directions, relaxing, breathing, surrendering.[4]

6. Observe all the transitions—the pause between the breaths, the gaps between thought, the levels of relaxation, transitions between feeling fully awake to dreaming to the darkness of deep sleep and beyond. Begin to notice when you are entering the hypnagogic state; see how long you can hover there without falling into sleep.

7. At the end of each practice, let awareness rest in the heart for several minutes. The heart is said to be one of the portals to freedom. You will know when to come out. Swami Veda taught that when the body releases a sigh, it's time to come out. Imagine that you are following prana to its source and that the Goddess Yoga Nidra is supporting you. She is supporting every breath, guiding you into the innermost cave of the heart. Rest in that cave.

8. Only your practice can lead you beyond this point. Listen to your intuition, your inner teacher. Research and read the texts, many of which you will find listed in the bibliography of this book. Sit with trusted teachers. Do research about teachers and lineages to identify those who have harmed others so you can make informed decisions. Ask teachers to explain where the teachings they share come from so you can do your own exploration.

9. Connect and share with your like-minded friends who are also interested in deepening these practices. Have them join you in sadhana so you can share experiences.

10. Experiment with the centers associated with the states of consciousness: the third eye (waking state), the throat center (dreaming state), the heart center (deep sleep), and deeper in the heart center (turiya).

All in all, the pathway to freedom is a journey that is never complete. We keep clearing the way with each practice and each breath. Every time we remember the lessons from our practices, we heal another part of ourselves.

Once we know what has healed and helped us, we can humbly share that with the world. And from that place of true embodiment, devotion, and love, we can share powerfully. Enlightenment is not a static state, so keep practicing, learning, and experimenting; no matter how abundant the fruits from your practice are, there is always more to be revealed.

May we know our true power
May we connect with the light within
May we be guided by our inner teacher
May we be a blessing to the world

Acknowledgments

My deepest gratitude and love:

To my beloved Harley, who unconditionally supported, loved, and held me while I spent days away from home or in my "cave" writing.

To my late father, Frederick Stanley, who taught me the value of waking up early, telling time by looking at the sun, and knowing that I was not defined by someone else's perceptions.

To my mother, Janice, for her unconditional love and unending support.

To my family—Harold, Brenda, Fred, Baron, Dane, Karen, Wendy, Sammy, Katie, Andrew, Barrett, and Alison.

To all those from whom I have learned so much over the years, especially Yogarupa Rod Stryker, Pandit Rajmani Tigunait, Swami Veda Bharati, Uma Dinsmore-Tuli, Gary Kraftsow, Dr. Richard Miller, Rolf Sovik, and Laura Amazzone.

To those who saw the future—the psychic at Elixir, Kat Alexander, and Kenneth Alexander.

To my dear sister Chanti Tacoronte-Perez for having the spirit to explore, cut cords, and create. Rosa and Louise are proud.

To my friends who cheered me on, inspired, and believed in me—Megan Monahan, Gina Gomez, Licia Morelli, Kim Krans, Michelle Cassandra Johnson, Mary Bruce, Katie Silcox, the community at Sacred Chill West Atlanta, Devon Craig, Heather Story, Suze Yalof Schwartz, Kelly Love Ross, Kate Northrup, Light Watkins, Dr. Gail Parker, and Danielle LaPorte.

To Jessica Levine for her help, her heart, and her eyes.

To my editor at Shambhala Publications, Sarah Stanton, for finding me. I still have your card on my altar.

To my agent, Dana Newman, for saying yes without hesitation.

To my illustrator, Maggie Lochtenberg, for a true connection with nature and spirit.

To the master of stick figures, Adam Grossi.

To those who supported me in my work and yoga trainings—Sari Gelzer, Crystal Higgins, Natalie Backman, Chris Johnson, Liesl Maggiore, April D'Aguilar, and Shivani Mehta.

To those who offered their valuable time, wisdom, and words—Octavia Raheem, Dr. Gail Parker, Dr. Dean Radin, Uma Dinsmore-Tuli, PhD, John Vosler, Chanti Tacoronte-Perez, Sonia Gibson, and Nkechi Njaka. I appreciate you.

Appendix

SCHOOLS OF YOGA NIDRA

iRest

Developed by Richard Miller, PhD, a world-renowned spiritual author, yogic scholar, researcher, and clinical psychologist, iRest combines traditional yogic practice with Western psychology and neuroscience. It has been used in numerous research studies addressing PTSD and trauma.

Himalayan Tradition

This tradition and lineage, known best for the "sixty-one points" and "seventy-five breaths" practices, has been popularized in the West by Swami Rama, Pandit Rajmani Tigunait, Swami Veda Bharati, and Rolf Sovic. Swami Rama was taught yogic sleep by the Mother Teacher, or Mataji.

ParaYoga Nidra

Developed by Yogarupa Rod Stryker and based on the Himalayan tradition, ParaYoga Nidra focuses on five modalities of practice: healing, transformation, sankalpa, transcendence, and accessing the timeless wisdom of the sages.

The Integrative Amrit Method of Yoga Nidra

Amrit and Kamini Desai, who developed the I AM method, describe it as a "powerful tool to master the inner dimension of life. A powerful sleep-based meditation technique that allows you to access the deepest state of meditation effortlessly."

Total Yoga Nidra

Total Yoga Nidra is a term developed 2010 by Dr. Uma Dinsmore-Tuli and Nirlipta Tuli, cofounders of the Yoga Nidra Network. TYN approach to sharing Yoga Nidra is post-lineage, decolonized, creative, and spontaneously responsive. Each Total Yoga Nidra is uniquely cocreated in response to the needs of the listeners and respectful of natural rhythms, locations, and cycles.

Bihar Tradition

This tradition focuses on the progressive, systematic relaxation of the body and mind using methods like the rotation of consciousness, visualization, symbols, pairs of opposites, and focus on the breath. It was one of the first lineages to popularize the practice of yoga nidra in the West.

YOGA POSES AND SEQUENCES FOR YOGA NIDRA

Describing yoga poses in depth is beyond the scope of this book. If you are looking for a resource for poses, sequences, and possible contraindications, you can check out books like *Wheelchair Yoga* by Jerri Lincoln; *Yoga for Wellness: Healing with the Timeless Teachings of Viniyoga* by Gary Kraftsow; *Yoga: Ancient Heritage, Tomorrow's Vision* by Indu Arora; *Yoni Shakti: A Woman's Guide to Power and Freedom through Yoga and Tantra* by Uma Dinsmore-Tuli; and *Yoga as Medicine: The Yogic Prescription for Health and Healing* by Timothy McCall, MD.

Yoga Poses

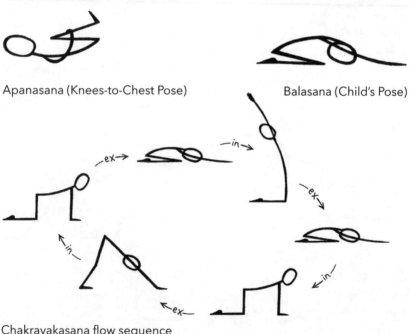

Apanasana (Knees-to-Chest Pose)

Balasana (Child's Pose)

Chakravakasana flow sequence
(Cat-Cow Flow)

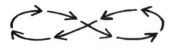

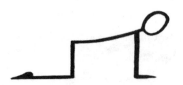

Figure Eights in Table-Top Position

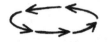

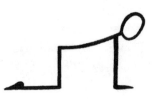

Hip Circles in Table-Top Position
(move hips)

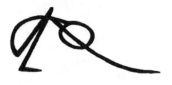

Malasana (Garland Pose)

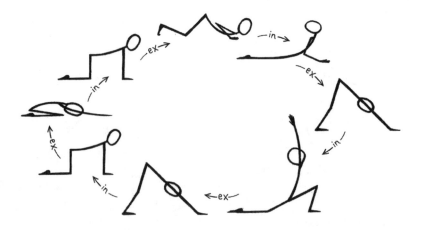

Moon Salutations

Salamba Sarvangasana
(Supported Shoulderstand)–
contraindicated if you have high
blood pressure, headaches, or a
neck injury, or if you are pregnant

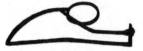

Paschimottanasana
(Seated Forward Bend)

Makarasana (Crocodile Pose)–
contraindicated if you have back pain
or are pregnant

Savasana (Corpse Pose)

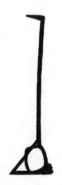

Sirsasana (Headstand)–
contraindicated if you have high
blood pressure or a neck injury

Sequences

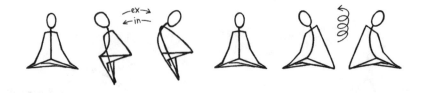

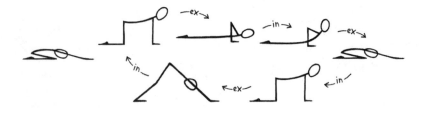

5X

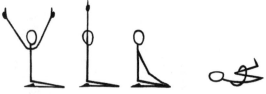

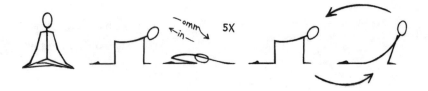

27 KAPALABHATI 3X

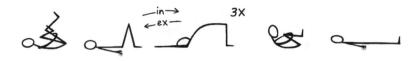

3X

−ex→
←in−

5X

−in→
←ex−

ROLL UP

SEED MANTRAS

GAM (pronounced *gum*) is a bija mantra of Ganesha, the grounding, healing destroyer of obstacles.

HAM (pronounced *hum*) activates prana, tejas, and *pitta* (the Ayurvedic dosha associated with fire and water elements; translated as "that which cooks"). Do not use it with nyasa practice without first consulting a knowledgeable teacher.

HRIM (pronounced *hreem*) is a bija mantra related to the sun and the planet of the heart, as well as to *hridaya* (the spiritual heart center). It is said to activate the heart on all levels—physical, energetic, and spiritual.

KRIM (pronounced *kreem*) is the bija mantra of Kali, the goddess of time and transformation.

LAM (pronounced *lum*) is a mantra associated with the earth element and the root chakra.

AUM (pronounced *aum*) is the mantra that represents the whole of the universe and the states of consciousness. It is the seed sound of energy and vitality, the sound of creation and the higher self.

SAUH (pronounced *sauha*) encourages the blissful nectar of soma to flow from the crown of the head to the heart center.

SRIM (pronounced *shreem*) relates to the moon and has a soothing effect on the mind. It is also the seed mantra of Lakshmi, the goddess of abundance. It is a perfect mantra to express our faith that the Goddess can hold, support, and nurture us, allowing our blissful and radiant natures to shine.

VAM (pronounced *vum*) connects us to the water element and the second chakra.

MANTRAS

A mantra is "revealed sound" and cannot be understood until the meaning is revealed through practice. The following descriptions provide the essence of the mantras rather than direct translations. Feel free to research the mantras further and do the practices to connect to what resonates with you. For a detailed look at mantras and pronunciation, see Sheela Bringi's Sacred Sound Lab (www.sacredsoundlab.com).

Gayatri Mantra

This mantra connects us to the radiance of Divine light. It is said to illuminate the singer and purify the listener.

> OM BHUR BHUVAH SWAH
>
> TAT-SAVITUR VAREÑYAM
>
> BHARGO DEVASYA DHĪMAHI
>
> DHIYO YONAH PRACHODAYĀT

May the light of consciousness that illuminates all the worlds sustain, inspire, and awaken me with its radiance.

Maha Mritjunjaya

This is a healing and nurturing mantra to awaken our internal healing forces.

> OM, TRYAMBAKAM YAJĀMAHE
>
> SUGANDHIM PUSTI-VARDHANAM
>
> URVĀ-RUKAMIVA BANDHANĀN
>
> MRTYOR-MUKSĪYA MĀ'MRTĀT

I meditate on, and surrender myself to, the Divine Being who embodies the power of will, the power of knowledge, and the power of action. I pray to the Divine Being who manifests in the form of fragrance in the flower of life and is the eternal nourisher of the plant of life. Like a skillful gardener, may the Lord of Life disentangle me from the binding forces of my physical, psychological, and spiritual foes. May the Lord of Immortality residing within free me from death, decay, and sickness and unite me with immortality.

Translation from the Himalayan Institute

Ratri Suktum Verse 10

Remember the story of Brahma singing praises to the Goddess Yoga Nidra to awaken Vishnu? This verse is part of that hymn. Take a moment to chant it in the moonlight when you need a cooling, calm, nurturing presence. *Saumya* means gentle in action; pearl-like; moonlike; evoking the qualities of purity, tranquility, and peacefulness.

SAUMYĀ SAUMYĀTARĀŚEṢĀ

SAUMYEBHYAS TVATI SUNDARI

PARĀPARĀṆĀṂ PARAMĀ

TVAMEVA PARAMESHVARĪ

You are beauty and more beauty. You are the most beautiful among all of the saumya things. You are Parameshwari, the Supreme Goddess beyond all things near and far.[1]

Shiva Sankalpa Sukta Refrain

This is a refrain from the Shiva Sankalpa Sukta. It is said to hold the benefits of the six verses that comprise the entire mantra and is perfect for those who cannot or do not have time to memorize the full mantra. The mantra in its entirety invites the mind to follow a flow of thought that is in aligned with our highest purpose and dharma.[2]

TAN ME MANAHA SHIVA SANKALPAM ATSU

May my mind be filled with auspicious thoughts.

PRANAYAMA

Bhramari Breath (Humming of the Bees)

This type of breathing soothes the nervous system and calms the mind.

This is a simplified version to get you started. Sit in a comfortable posture, and close your eyes. Inhale and exhale through your nose, with your lips closed and your upper and lower teeth touching. Make a low-pitched humming sound, much like a hive of bees, as you exhale. Feel the vibration of the hum vibrating through your teeth, tongue, and brain. Feel it clearing and calming your whole system. (3–5 minutes)

Chandra Bhedana (Moon-Piercing Breath)

This pranayama activates the lunar channel and is cooling to both the body and the mind.

Hold your right nostril closed as you inhale through the left; now hold the left nostril closed while you exhale through the right. Inhale, left; exhale, right again. Continue inhaling only through your left nostril and exhaling through your right. Visualize a small moon floating near your left nostril, and feel as though you are inhaling the vapors of the moon. Feel the healing and cooling power of the moon spreading through your entire body and mind. (3 minutes)

Circular Breathing

This type of breathing brings a sense of peace, calm, and inner stillness.

Bring awareness to your navel. Watch it rise on the inhalation and fall on the exhalation. Witness your breath; let go of controlling or judging it. (1 minute)

Begin to smooth out any rough edges that you notice in your breath; let the flow become smooth and free. (1 minute)

Notice the pause between the inhalation and the exhalation.

Imagine that you can draw a circle of moonlight in front of you from the floor to the ceiling.

Feel the gap between the in-breath and the out-breath gradually become smaller as you observe your breath traveling around the circle of moonlight with no pauses, gaps, or breaks.

You can reduce your breathing capacity to about half or one-third (or take slightly shorter breaths) as you witness your breath traveling around the circle in an unbroken, even stream. Feel a sense of peace and bliss unfolding and increasing with each breath. (2 minutes)

Diaphragmatic Breathing

This pranayama cultivates breath awareness and activates your parasympathetic nervous system, or your body's rest-and-digest state. It is the foundation of cultivating effortless breathing.

For this simplified version, sit in a chair or lie in Savasana (Corpse Pose). Bring awareness to your body as you breathe. Notice the area around your belly: allow it to relax, and let go of trying to suck it in. As you breathe in, let your belly expand, and as you breathe out, let it fall. As you inhale, your navel rises; as you exhale, it moves closer to the spine. Let your breath become smooth, silent, and even in length on the inhale and exhale, without a pause between the inhale and exhale. (5 minutes)

Nadi Shodhana (Alternate Nostril Breathing)

This type of breathing balances the mind and the energies in the body.

Place your right hand in Vishnu mudra. Use your right thumb to close off your right nostril and rest the fourth and fifth fingers on your left nostril (so you can close that nostril when needed). Inhale through your left nostril; lift your thumb from the right nostril, close the left with your fingers, and exhale through your right nostril. Now inhale through the right nostril, lift your fingers from the left, press the right nostril closed with your thumb, and exhale from the left.

Continue in this pattern: Inhale, left; exhale, right. Inhale, right; exhale, left. Inhale, left; exhale, right. Inhale, right; exhale, left; and so on. (5 minutes)

1:2 Breathing

An exhalation twice the length of the inhalation (i.e., inhale four counts, exhale eight counts) activates the parasympathetic nervous system and promotes relaxation.

Begin by noticing your breath flowing in and out. Begin to count as you inhale; start with counting to 4 if it feels comfortable. As you exhale, double the length of the inhalation. If you inhaled for 4 counts, exhale for 8 counts. Find a breath ratio that works for you—do not strain. (3 minutes)

Prana Dharana (Vital Energy Concentration)

This is a practice of directing, collecting, and building prana in a particular place.

Find a comfortable and stable seated posture for this simple version of the practice. Notice the flow of breath as it enters your nostrils. Notice that the temperature of your breath as it enters your nostrils is cool; as it exits the nostrils, it is warmer. Be aware that prana is riding on your breath. Imagine you can feel, see, or sense light riding along with the breath. As you inhale, light travels simultaneously through both nostrils to the third eye, where the two streams of light meet. As you exhale, light or prana moves from the third eye back out through both nostrils. See yourself following this inverted V of light through both nostrils to the third eye and back out through both nostrils as you continue to build and collect light at the third eye.

Once you have collected prana at this point, it can be directed elsewhere in your body, such as to the heart or navel center. (9 times)

MEDITATIONS

Apana Vayu Meditation *3 minutes*

Grounds and stabilizes

Sit in a meditation posture. Bring your attention to the base of your spine and visualize a blue, downward-pointing triangle there. As you breathe out, see a bolt of lightning moving from the apex of this triangle into the earth. Feel this stabilizing and grounding you.[3]

Shusumna Meditation *10 minutes*

Develops sensitivity to prana and clears energetic blocks

Sit in a meditation posture. Allow yourself to cultivate a sense of effortlessness. Imagine that there is a clear glass tube that runs through the center of your spine. Bring your attention to the base of your spine. As you breathe in, imagine, feel, or sense that the breath travels though the tube from the base of your spine to the crown of your head. You might see the breath as light, smoke from an incense stick, or even water rising in the tube. On your exhalation, feel the breath travel down through the tube from the crown of your head to the base of your spine. As you feel the breath move up the spine on the inhale, hear the sound SO. As you feel or see the breath descend from the crown of your head to the base of your spine, hear the sound HAM. Continue to witness breath ascending through the glass tube on the inhale and descending on the exhale as you hear the mantra SO HAM.

SUSTAINED AWARENESS PRACTICES

Dream Stone Practice (Overnight Practice)

For this practice, you will need a small crystal or stone. When you are ready to sleep, hold the crystal or stone in your nondominant hand.

As you hold the stone, take a moment to be present to your breath. Repeat your chosen sankalpa silently to yourself; for example, *I am worthy of love.*

Now set the intention that you will not drop or let go of the crystal through the course of the night. The key to this practice is the feeling of effortlessness. Don't get caught up in the idea of doing it right—it's a practice!

Any time you awake during the night, remember the crystal, or if you have dropped it, place it back in your hand and repeat your sankalpa once to yourself. Go back to sleep. Each time you wake up or lose the crystal, repeat the process.

This practice helps to develop your awareness of the dreaming state and helps you to cultivate awareness of the transitions and to stay awake and aware during yoga nidra practices.

108 Countdown (Overnight Countdown)

This practice is one of my favorites. When I did it for thirty days, it changed my relationship with deep relaxation and helped me to resist falling asleep in the practice.

As you go to sleep, begin to count down from 108 all the way to zero.[4] Watch yourself fall asleep. Remember the number where you left off, and when you wake up during the night, continue the countdown from that number. Repeat this during the night, maintaining the countdown until you get to zero. If you reach zero before it is time to wake up, begin to count up to 108 again.

Let go of trying to get to zero or back up to 108. That is not the point of the practice. This is not a practice to try to compete with yourself. Let go of getting it right—otherwise you may be up all night. You are just training yourself to stay awake and aware while you relax effort. When you are ready to wake up to start your day, give yourself 5 minutes to freewrite in your dream journal.

If you have insomnia or any sleep disorder, please consult with your physician before trying these practices. Limit your use of them to two or three consecutive days at a time until you understand how they affect you.

Glossary

abhyanga The Ayurvedic practice of massaging the body with oil. See page 105.

altar A sacred place to make offerings, prayers, or intentions. See page 72.

ancestor Any person from whom one is descended; however, some would also consider the earth to be an ancestor. See page 56.

bija mantra (seed sound) A single-syllable sound that affects a chakra or the subtle body. See page 6.

biofeedback Electronic monitoring of the body's involuntary systems for the purpose of self-regulation. See page 20.

biohacking Incremental lifestyle changes that optimize health and well-being. See page 1.

Devi Mahatmya The primary text of the Shakta tradition, which is also part of the Markandeya Purana. See page 17.

Devi Suktam A hymn praising the Divine Mother and her many powers that uphold the universe. See page 22.

epigenetics The study of external modifications to DNA that turn genes on or off. See page 60.

freewriting The act of processing experience through writing—quickly without concern for sentence structure, grammar, or spelling—to deepen understanding and cultivate memory and retentive power (*smirti*). See page 8.

guru chakra The energy center that resides between the eyebrows and the crown of the head; a portal to the inner teacher. See page 163.

Himalayan tradition A lineage that extends back thousands of years and is rooted in the wisdom of Patanjali's Yoga Sutras and tantra. See page 19.

householder A lay spiritual practitioner living in the world, as opposed to an ashram or hermitage, whose primary concerns relate to the upkeep of his or her home, family, or career. See page 5.

hridaya The spiritual heart center, which in some traditions is said to be the seat of consciousness. See page 42.

koshas Layers, or casings, of consciousness that move from the gross to the subtle and cover the light of the soul. See page 24.

mantra A sound that guides and protects the mind and that effects change on the level of the subtle body. See page 6.

marma points Ayurvedic energy pathways for healing the body, mind, and consciousness; similar to acupuncture points in Traditional Chinese Medicine. See page 123.

Mataji (also known as "Mother Teacher") The sage who taught Swami Rama the practice of "sleepless sleep." See page 20.

mauna The practice of silence. See page 132.

mudra (seal) A hand gesture or body posture (such as maha mudra) that channel the body's energy flow. See page 79.

nidra To sleep or to draw forth from the void (*ni* means "void," and *dru* means "to draw forth"). See page 1.

Nidra Shakti The power of sleep, or the power of repose. See page 48.

nirvikalpa "No thought" of the difference between one's spirit and the Divine. See page 35.

nyasa To place, plant, or install. See page 126.

parasympathetic nervous system The body's healing, rejuvenating system, also known as the rest-and-digest system. See page 62.

post-traumatic stress disorder (PTSD) A psychiatric disorder that can occur in people who have experienced or witnessed a traumatic event. See page 19.

prana A vital life force that animates the body and mind. See page 16.

pranayama Breath control; the practice that brings awareness to the energetic body, the fourth limb of yoga. It is both the restraint of prana and the expansion of prana. See page 6.

pratyahara The withdrawal of the senses, moving from the external to the internal; the fifth limb of yoga and a key element of any deep relaxation practice. See page 16.

pre-practices Preparatory exercises for deep relaxation or techniques that lead to the state of yoga nidra. See page 6.

race-based stress and trauma An injury resulting from the emotional pain that a person may feel after encounters with racism. See page 55.

radiance Light that is emitted or reflected. See page 2.

relaxation response The term coined by Herbert Benson, MD, in 1975 to describe the body's rest-and-digest state. See page 61.

rest Quiet, freedom from toil, refreshing ease, peace of mind or spirit; the result of yoga nidra practice. See page 2.

restorative yoga A form of yoga that uses props to support the body in relaxed and calming postures held for long periods of time. Although some restorative postures may be used in your yoga nidra nest, restorative yoga is not the same as yoga nidra. See page 56.

rewilding A holistic approach to living that returns you to your natural state through a connection with nature. See page 7.

rishis, rishikas The original seers of yoga. See page 2.

ritual An observance, ceremony, or way of doing something. See page 6.

sadhana Dedicated practice over time, spiritual discipline. See page 102.

sankalpa An awareness of and commitment to a heartfelt resolve that leads to your highest truth. See page 6.

saumya Gentleness in action; pearl-like, moonlike; evoking the qualities of purity, tranquility, and peacefulness. See page 149.

self-inquiry A process of bringing attention to one's innermost thoughts and inner awareness. See page 6.

shakti The feminine power of the Divine Mother or deity; cosmic vibration. See page 48.

siddhis Paranormal powers that arise from the practice of yoga; also said to be the obstacles to the path of yoga. See page 16.

smirti The power of retention and memory. See page 47.

social location Reflects the many intersections of our experience related to race, religion, age, physical size, sexual orientation, social class, and so on. Social location contributes not only to our understanding of the ways in which our major institutions work but also to our ability to access them. See page 71.

soma The nectar of devotion, bliss. See page 155.

sound baths A healing modality of meditative relaxation where musical instruments or the human voice is used to cocoon or bathe the participant in sound waves. See page 63.

states of consciousness Various conditions of awareness described in the Mandukya Upanishad, including waking, dreaming, deep sleep, and turiya. See page 3.

subtle body The subtle or energetic anatomy composed of the koshas, chakras, vayus, and so on. See page 24.

sympathetic nervous system The system responsible for the fight-or-flight response, when the body senses danger and releases hormones and chemicals to increase heart rate, breathing rate, blood pressure, metabolic rate, and blood flow to the muscles, preparing the body to either defend itself or escape. See page 62.

tantra The technology of energy management that includes practices for worldly and spiritual prosperity. See page 19.

tapas Austerity, heat; the heat, produced by the friction of practice, that has the power to transform. See page 168.

trauma Held tension, stress, and/or emotional energy stemming from distressing or overwhelming events in one's past. See page 51.

Upanishads The philosophical portion of the Vedas; the foundation of Vedanta and Jnana Yoga. See page 17.

vritti A wave or fluctuation. See page 134.

Yoga Sutras A collection of 196 Sanskrit aphorisms on the theory and practice of yoga that was compiled by the sage Patanjali. See page 16.

Notes

INTRODUCTION · YOGA NIDRA: BEYOND TECHNIQUE

1. CNRS, "A new discovery: How our memories stabilize while we sleep," ScienceDaily, October 18, 2019, www.sciencedaily.com /releases/2019/10/191018125514.htm.
2. Notes from Rod Stryker lecture, May 2017.
3. Sri Aurobindo, *The Life Divine*, p. 1065.

1 · THE MYSTERY OF YOGA NIDRA

1. My favorite definition of yoga is from Swami Veda Bharati, "Yoga is Samadhi." For more information, see https://www.parmarth.org/yoga /yoga-definition/.
2. Swami Veda Bharati, *Yoga Sutras of Patanjali, Volume 2*, p. 468.
3. Swami Veda Bharati, *Yoga Sutras of Patanjali, Volume 2*, p. 468.
4. Birch and Hargreaves, "Yoganidrā."
5. Birch and Hargreaves, "Yoganidrā."
6. Uma Dinsmore-Tuli, *Yoni Shakti*, loc. 1137 of 17420, Kindle.
7. Swami Veda Bharati, *My Experiments with Yoga Nidra*, loc. 114 of 316, Kindle.
8. Swami Rama, *Living with the Himalayan Masters*, loc. 1115 of 4462, Kindle.

9. The *Devimatyma*, which is also part of the *Markendeya Purana*, a Hindu text thought to have been written between the second and seventh century C.E. Sri Ravi Shankar, "Significance of Devi Stotra," The Art of Living (website), posted October 7, 2016, https://www.artofliving.org /wisdom/wssst/significance-of-devi-stotra.

10. Karline McLain, *India's Immortal Comic Books: Gods, Kings, and Other Heroes* (Bloomington: Indiana University Press, 2009), p. 91.

11. Birch and Hargreaves, "Yoganidrā."

12. Notes from the Masterclass with Neil deGrasse Tyson, "Teaches Scientific Thinking and Communication."

2 · THE JOURNEY THROUGH CONSCIOUSNESS

1. Elda and Irving Hartley, *Biofeedback*, presented by Elmer Green.

2. Green, "Biofeedback and Yoga," https://journals.sfu.ca/seemj/index. php/seemj/article/viewFile/265/228.

3. Green, "Biofeedback and Yoga."

4. Gay Luce and Ebik Peper, "Mind Over Body, Mind Over Mind," *New York Times*, September 12, 1971, https://www.nytimes.com/1971/09/12 /archives/mind-over-body-mind-over-mind-such-is-the-twin-promise-of. html.

5. Ned Herrmann, "What is the function of the various brainwaves?" Scientific American (website), December 22, 1997, https://www.scientific american.com/article/what-is-the-function-of-t-1997-12-22/.

6. Priyanka A. Abhang, Bharti W. Gawali, Suresh C. Mehrotra, "Technical Aspects of Brain Rhythms and Speech Parameters," in *Introduction to EEG- and Speech-Based Emotion Recognition* (London: Elsevier, 2016), pp. 51–79, https://www.sciencedirect.com/science/article/pii/ B9780128044902000038.

7. Walker, *Why We Sleep*, p. 44, Kindle.

8. Eric Suni, "Stages of Sleep," Sleep Foundation (website), August 14, 2020, https://www.sleepfoundation.org/articles/stages-of-sleep.

9. Robert Nilsson, "Pictures of the Brain's Activity during Yoga Nidra," HAA International Retreat Center at the Scandinavian Yoga and Meditation School. https://www.yogameditation.com/reading-room/pictures-of-the-brains-activity-during-yoga-nidra/.

10. For translations of the 4 states, see Swami Rama, *OM the Eternal Witness*, loc. 1695–97, Kindle.

11. Swami Lakshmanjoo, *Kashmir Shaivism: The Secret Supreme* (self-pub., Universal Shaiva Fellowship, 2015), loc. 2868 of 4824, Kindle.

12. Sri Ramanananda, *Tripura Rahasya: The Secret of the Supreme Goddess* (Bloomington, IN: World Wisdom, 2002), p. 59, Kindle.

13. Swami Rama, *OM the Eternal Witness*, loc. 1695–97, Kindle.

14. Stephen Parker, Swami Veda Bharati, Manuel Fernandez, "Defining Yoga-Nidra: Traditional Accounts, Physiological Research, and Future Directions," *International Journal of Yoga Therapy* 23, no. 1 (September 2013): https://pubmed.ncbi.nlm.nih.gov/24016819/.

15. Paul Brunton and Munagala Venkataramiah, *Conscious Immortality: Conversations with Sri Ramanasramam* (Tiruvannamalai, India: Sri Ramanasramam, 1984), loc. 1891 of 3534, Kindle.

16. From my Ayurvedic teacher Ragaia Belovarac of Blue Sage Ayurveda in Grass Valley, California.

17. Swami Lakshmanjoo, *The Manual for Self-Realization: 112 Meditations of the Vijnana Bhairava Tantra* (self-pub., Universal Shaiva Fellowship, 2015), loc. 8474–79, Kindle.

18. Walker, *Why We Sleep*, p. 232, Kindle.

19. Personal communication, email message to author, May 6, 2020.

20. Swami Lakshmanjoo, *Kashmir Shaivism*, loc. 2893 of 4824, Kindle.

21. Swami Veda Bharati, *Yoga Sutras of Patanjali, Volume 2*, p. 638.

22. Swami Lakshmanjoo, *Kashmir Shaivism*, loc. 1183 of 4824, Kindle.

23. Dinsmore-Tuli, *Yoni Shakti*, loc. 5150 of 17420, Kindle.

24. Cassandra Vieten et al., "Future Directions in Meditation Research: Recommendations for Expanding the Field of Contemplative Science." PLoS ONE 13, no. 11 (2018): e0205740. https://doi.org/10.1371/journal. pone.0205740.

25. Swami Veda Bharati, *Meditation: The Art and Science* (Los Angeles: SCB Distributors, 2008), p. 130, Kindle.

26. Swami Veda Bharati, *Yoga Sutras of Patanjali, Volume 2*, p. 752.

27. Personal communication, email message to author, February 17, 2020.

3 · WHAT DOES IT MEAN TO RELAX?

1. La Barre, *Issues in Your Tissues*, p. 110, Kindle.

2. Stankovic, "Transforming Trauma," 23–37.

3. Personal communication, phone call and email message to author, February 12, 2020.

4. Daniel Foor, "Rituals and Boundaries" (class lecture notes, April 12, 2020).

5. Personal communication with Octavia Raheem, email message to author, December 26, 2019.

6. Costa, Yetter, and DeSomer, "Intergenerational Transmission of Paternal Trauma," 11215–20.

7. Benson, *The Relaxation Response*, p. 7, Kindle.

8. Benson, *The Relaxation Response*, p. 10, Kindle.

9. Personal communication with John Vosler, email message to author, July 7, 2020.

10. I first learned this practice from Los Angeles–based yoga teacher Julian Walker, and then from Swami Veda Bharati. This practice combines the two.

11. Inspired by Swami Veda Bharati.

4 · THE HOUSEHOLDER'S FLOW

1. Groden, "How Many Americans Sleep with Their Smartphones," *Fortune*.
2. Easwaran, *Upanishads*, second ed., p. 6.
3. Devi, *Secret Power of Yoga*, p. 279, Kindle.
4. Northrup, *Do Less*, p. 155.
5. Tigunait, *The Practice of the Yoga Sutra*, p. 174.

5 · HOW TO PREPARE FOR YOGA NIDRA

1. Personal communication with Uma Dinsmore-Tuli, email message to author, February 5, 2020.

6 · PRACTICE ONE: GROUNDING AND STABILITY

1. Frawley, *Inner Tantric Yoga*, p. 99.
2. Frawley, *Yoga and Ayurveda*, loc. 2356 of 3223.

7 · PRACTICE TWO: WAVES OF AUM

1. Swami Veda Bharati, *Yoga Sutras of Patanjali, Volume 2*, p. 762.
2. Dvadashanta is traditionally taught as twelve fingers width away from hands, feet, base of spine, and crown of head.
3. Practice inspired by an experience with Swami Radha Bharati, August 12, 2018.
4. The nose is considered to be a microcosm of the chakra system and connected to shusumna. The tip of the nose corresponds to the base of the spine while the bridge relates to the third eye point. See Lad and Durve, *Marma Points of Ayurveda*, p. 100.

8 · PRACTICE THREE: DEEP RELAXATION, ESSENTIAL ACTIVATION

1. Michael Grady, "A Practice of 61-Points to Sharpen Concentration," Yoga International, https://yogainternational.com/article/view/a-practice-of-61-points-to-sharpen-concentration.
2. Swami Veda Bharati, *Yoga Sutras of Patanjali, Volume 2*, p. 763.
3. This is a video that we used in our training when we were unable to meet due to the pandemic. The students really loved it, and it gave them a very powerful experience of being under the stars: https://www.youtube.com/watch?time_continue=1&v=1-YOlGoKxeM&feature=emb_title&ab_channel=4KUltraHDVideo.

9 · PRACTICE FOUR: THE LIGHT OF INNER KNOWING

1. Frawley, Ranade, and Lele, *Ayurveda and Marma Therapy*, loc. 1973 of 2939, Kindle.
2. Maheshkumar Kuppusamy, Dilara Kamaldeen, Ravishankar Pitani, and Julius Amaldas, "Immediate Effects of Bhramari Pranayama on Resting Cardiovascular Parameters in Healthy Adolescents," *Journal of Clinical and Diagnostic Research* 10, no. 5 (2016): CC17–19. doi:10.7860/JCDR/2016/19202.7894.
3. Swami Lokeswarananda, *Chandogya Upanishad* (Roseville, MN: Ramakrishna Mission Institute of Culture, 2017), verse 8.1.2.

11 · PRACTICE SIX: INTO THE VOID

1. Definition of Mahavakya provided by Easwaran, *Upanishads*, Book 1, p. 340.

CONCLUSION · THE TRUE SECRET TO FREEDOM

1. Personal notes from Gary Kraftsow's presentation at the Heart-Mind Retreat in Austin, TX, December 2019.
2. Joe Dispenza, "The Habit of Your New Self," Dr. Joe Dispenza (blog), March 30, 2018, https://blog.drjoedispenza.com/blog/change/the-habit-of-your-new-self.
3. Tigunait, *Shiva Sutra*, p. 3.
4. This is pratyahara. Drop into a two-pronged awareness of watching yourself, and be aware of the one who is witnessing you watch yourself.

APPENDIX

1. Tantroktam Rātrisūktam: Praise of the Goddess Night, http://www.babachants.com/TantroktamRatrisuktamFull.pdf.
2. See Swami Tejomayanandana, *Divinising the Mind*, p. 5; Swami Veda Bharati, *Shiva Sankalpa Sukta*, p. 4.
3. Frawley, *Yoga and Ayurveda*, loc. 2360 of 3223, Kindle.
4. Bonnasse, *Yoga Nidra Meditation*, loc. 1404 of 2678, Kindle.

Bibliography

Abhang, Priyanka A., Bharti W. Gawali, and Suresh C. Mehrotra. "Technical Aspects of Brain Rhythms and Speech Parameters." In *Introduction to EEG- and Speech-Based Emotion Recognition*, 51–79. London: Academic Press, 2016.

American Institute of Vedic Studies. "The Original Teachings of Yoga: From Patanjali Back to Hiranyagarbha." December 19, 2019. www.vedanet.com/the-original-teachings-of-yoga-from-patanjali-back-to-hiranyagarbha.

American Psychiatric Association. "What Is Posttraumatic Stress Disorder?" Last reviewed January 2020. www.psychiatry.org/patients-families/ptsd/what-is-ptsd.

Arora, Indu. *Yoga: Ancient Heritage, Tomorrow's Vision*. Self-published, Yog Sadhna, 2019.

Arya, Pandit Usharbudh. *Yoga-Sutras of Patanjali with the Exposition of Vyasa*, vol. 1. Honesdale, PA: Himalayan International Institute of Yoga Science and Philosophy, 1986.

Aurobindo, Sri. *Savatri: A Legend and a Symbol*. Twin Lakes, WI: Lotus Press, 1995.

———. *The Life Divine*. Pondichery, India: Lotus Press, 2010.

Bear, Mark F., Barry W. Connors, and Michael A. Paradiso. *Neuroscience: Exploring the Brain*. 4th ed. Philadelphia, PA: Wolters Kluwer, 2016.

Benson, Herbert. *The Relaxation Response*. New York: Quill, 2001.

Bharati, Swami Veda. *My Experiments with Yoga Nidra*. Rishikesh, India: Himalayan Yoga Publications Trust, 2014.

———. *Shiva Sankalpa Sukta*. Rishikesh, India: Himalayan Yoga Publications Trust, 2007.

———. "Shiva Sankalpa Sukta," Ahymsin. February 26, 2011. https://ahymsin .org/main/swami-veda-bharati/shiva-sankalpa-sukta.html.

———. "Yoga Nidra No. 1." Lecture, 1:00:34. Filmed 2009. Posted by Panditji Tejomaya, November 30, 2015. www.youtube.com/watch?v=A_ee3q9cl1A.

———. *Yoga Sutras of Patanjali*. 2 vols. Honesdale, PA: Himalayan International Institute of Yoga Science and Philosophy, 1984.

———. *Yogi in the Lab*. Rishikesh, India: Himalayan Yoga Publications Trust, 2006.

Birch, Jason, and Jacqueline Hargreaves. "Yoganidrā: An Understanding of the History and Context." The Luminescent (website). January 6, 2015. https://www.theluminescent.org/2015/01/yoganidra.html.

Bonnasse, Pierre. *Yoga Nidra Meditation: The Sleep of the Sages*. Rochester, VT: Inner Traditions, 2017.

Boyd, Doug. *Swami: Encounters with Modern Mystics*. Honesdale, PA: Himalayan Institute Press, 2007.

Brown, Emery N., Ralph Lydic, and Nicholas D. Schiff. "General Anesthesia, Sleep, and Coma." *New England Journal of Medicine* 363, no. 27 (2010): 2638–50. https://pubmed.ncbi.nlm.nih.gov/21190458.

Carter, Robert. "Race-Based Traumatic Stress." *Psychiatric Times*, December 1, 2006, www.psychiatrictimes.com/race-based-traumatic-stress.

Cashford, Jules. *The Moon: Myth and Image*. New York: Four Walls Eight Windows, 2002.

Chaturvedi, B. K. *The Supreme Mother Goddess Durga: Mythological References, Tales of Glory, Hymns, Orisons and Devotional Songs*. Delhi, India: Diamond Pocket Books, 2003.

Chinmayananda, Swami. *Taittiriya Upanishad*. Mumbai, India: Chinmaya Prakashan, 2013.

Coburn, Thomas B. *Devi Mahatmya: The Crystallization of the Goddess Tradition*. Delhi, India: Motilal Banarsidass, 2002.

Costa, Dora L., Noelle Yetter, and Heather DeSomer. "Intergenerational Transmission of Paternal Trauma among US Civil War ex-POWs." *Proceedings of the National Academy of Sciences of the United States of America* 115, no. 44 (2018): 11215–20. doi.org/10.1073/pnas.1803630115.

Dale, Cyndi. *The Subtle Body: An Encyclopedia of Your Energetic Anatomy.* Boulder, CO: Sounds True, 2009.

Debroy, Bibek, and Dipavali Debroy. *The Markandeya Purana.* Delhi, India: Books for All, 2016.

Devi, Nischala Joy. *The Secret Power of Yoga: A Woman's Guide to the Heart and Spirit of the Yoga Sutras.* New York: Three Rivers Press, 2007.

DiNardo, Kelly, and Amy Pearce-Hayden. *Living the Sutras: A Guide to Yoga Wisdom beyond the Mat.* Boulder, CO: Shambhala Publications, 2018.

Dinsmore-Tuli, Uma. Total Yoga Nidra Workshop. Lecture notes. Phoenix, AZ, March 2018.

———. *Yoni Shakti: A Woman's Guide to Power and Freedom through Yoga and Tantra.* London: YogaWords, 2014.

Dispenza, Joe. *Breaking the Habit of Being Yourself: How to Lose Your Mind and Create a New One.* Reprint, Carlsbad, CA: Hay House, 2013.

———. *Evolve Your Brain: The Science of Changing Your Mind.* Deerfield Beach, FL: Health Communications, Inc., 2007.

Easwaran, Eknath. *The Upanishads.* 2nd ed. 2 vols. Tomales, CA: Nilgiri Press, 2007.

———, trans. *The Bhagavad Gita.* 2nd ed. Tomales, CA: Nilgiri Press, 2007. See esp. chap. 2 v. 69.

Emerson, David. *Trauma-Sensitive Yoga in Therapy: Bringing the Body into Treatment.* New York: W. W. Norton, 2015.

Fasta, Elizabeth, and Delphine Collin Vézinab. "Historical Trauma, Race-Based Trauma, and Resilience of Indigenous Peoples: A Literature Review." *First Peoples Child and Family Review* 14, no. 1 (2019): 166–81.

Frawley, David. *Inner Tantric Yoga: Working with the Universal Shakti.* Twin Lakes, WI: Lotus Press, 2008.

———. *Mantra Yoga and Primal Sound: Secret of Seed (Bija) Mantras*. Twin Lakes, WI: Lotus Press, 2010.

———. *Soma in Yoga and Ayurveda: The Power of Rejuvenation and Immortality*. Twin Lakes, WI: Lotus Press, 2012.

———. *Vedic Yoga: The Path of the Rishi*. Twin Lakes, WI: Lotus Press, 2014.

———. *Yoga and Ayurveda: Self-Healing and Self-Realization*. Twin Lakes, WI: Lotus Press, 1999.

Frawley, David, Subhash Ranade, and Avinash Lele. *Ayurveda and Marma Therapy: Energy Points in Yogic Healing*. Twin Lakes, WI: Lotus Press, 2003.

Gorvett, Zarvia. "What You Can Learn from Einstein's Quirky Habits." Future, June 12, 2017. www.bbc.com/future/article/20170612-what-you -can-learn-from-einsteins-quirky-habits.

Green, Elmer. "Biofeedback and Yoga." *Subtle Energies & Energy Medicine* 10, no. 1 (1974): 46–52.

Green, Elmer and Alyce. *Beyond Biofeedback*. New York: Delacorte Press, 1977.

Groden, Claire. "Here's How Many Americans Sleep with Their Smartphones." *Fortune*. June 29, 2015. https://fortune.com/2015/06/29/sleep -banks-smartphones.

Hartley, Elda and Irving, producers. *Biofeedback: The Yoga of the West*. Presented by Elmer Green. Cos Cob, CT: Hartley Films, 1975.

Hartman, Courtney. "Exploring the Experiences of Women with Complex Trauma and the Practice of iRest–Yoga Nidra." PhD diss., California Institute of Integral Studies, 2015. https://www.irest.org/sites/default /files/iRest-and-Women-with-Complex-Trauma.pdf.

Iyengar, B. K. S. *Light on the Yoga Sutras of Patanjali*. London: Thorsons, 2002.

Jagadiswaranda, Swami. *Devi Mahatmyam: Glory of the Divine Mother*. Madras, India: Sri Ramakrishna Math, 1953.

Kālī, Devadatta. *In Praise of the Goddess: The Devimahatmya and Its Meaning*. Berwick, ME: Nicolas-Hays, Inc., 2003.

Kirkinis, Katherine, Alex L. Pieterse, Christina Martin, Alex Agiliga, and Amanda Brownell. "Racism, Racial Discrimination, and Trauma: A Systematic Review of the Social Science Literature." *Ethnicity & Health*, August 30, 2018, 1–21.

Kolk, Bessel van der. *The Body Keeps the Score: Brain, Mind, and Body in the Healing of Trauma*. New York: Penguin Books, 2014.

Kraftsow, Gary. Heart-Mind Retreat. Lecture notes. Austin, TX, December 2019.

———. *Yoga for Wellness: Healing with the Timeless Teachings of Viniyoga*. New York: Penguin, 1999.

La Barre, Denise. *Issues in Your Tissues: Heal Body and Emotion from the Inside Out*. Haiku, HI: Healing Catalyst Press, 2010.

Lad, Vasant, and Anisha Durve. *Marma Points of Ayurveda: The Energy Pathways for Healing Body, Mind, and Consciousness with a Comparison to Traditional Chinese Medicine*. Albuquerque, NM: The Ayurvedic Press, 2015.

Lasater, Judith Hanson. *Restore and Rebalance: Yoga for Deep Relaxation*. Boulder, CO: Shambhala, 2017.

Lincoln, Jerri. *Wheelchair Yoga*. Prescott, AZ: Ralston Store Publishing, 2012.

Luders, Eileen, Arthur W. Toga, Natasha Lepore, and Christian Gaser, "The Underlying Anatomical Correlates of Long-Term Meditation: Larger Hippocampal and Frontal Volumes of Gray Matter. *NeuroImage* 45, no. 3 (2009): 672–78. doi.org/10.1016/j.neuroimage.2008.12.061.

Lutz, Antoine, Lawrence L. Greischar, Nancy B. Rawlings, Matthieu Ricard, and Richard J. Davidson. "Long-Term Meditators Self-Induce High-Amplitude Gamma Synchrony during Mental Practice." *Proceedings of the National Academy of Sciences of the United States of America* 101, no. 46 (2004): 16369–73. doi.org/10.1073/pnas.0407401101.

Maharshi, Bhagavan Sri Ramana. *Self-Enquiry (Vichara Sangraham) of Bhagavan Sri Ramana Maharshi*. Translated by T. M. P. Mahadevan. Tamil Nadu, India: Sri Ramanasramam, 1971.

"Mandukya Upanishad and Yoga: Twelve Verses on OM Mantra." Traditional Yoga and Meditation of the Himalayan Masters. Accessed July 27, 2020. www.swamij.com/mandukya-upanishad.htm.

McCall, Timothy. *Yoga as Medicine: The Yogic Prescription for Health and Healing*. New York: Bantam Books, 2007.

Muktibodhanda, Swami. *Swara Yoga*. Bihar, India: Bihar School of Yoga, 1999.

Northrup, Kate. *Do Less: A Revolutionary Approach to Time and Energy Management for Ambitious Women*. New York: Hay House, 2019.

Ozdemir, Ahmet, and Serdar Saritas. "Effect of Yoga Nidra on the Self-Esteem and Body Image of Burn Patients." *Complementary Therapies in Clinical Practice* 35 (2019): 86–91. doi.org/10.1016/j.ctcp.2019.02.002.

Pence, Pamela G., Lori S. Katz, Cristi Huffman, and Geta Cojucar. "Delivering Integrative Restoration–Yoga Nidra Meditation (iRest®) to Women with Sexual Trauma at a Veteran's Medical Center: A Pilot Study." *International Journal of Yoga Therapy* 24 (2014): 53–62.

Polanco-Roman Lillian, Ashley Danies, and Deidre M. Anglin. "Racial Discrimination as Race-Based Trauma, Coping Strategies and Dissociative Symptoms among Emerging Adults." *Psychological Trauma* 8, no. 5 (2016): 609–17. doi.org/10.1037/tra0000125.

Rama, Swami. *Exercises for Joints and Glands: Simple Movement to Enhance Your Well-Being*. 2nd ed. Honesdale, PA: Himalayan Institute Press, 2007.

———. *Living with the Himalayan Masters*. Allahabad, India: Himalayan Institute India, 1999.

———. *OM the Eternal Witness: Secrets of the Mandukya Upanishad*. Twin Lakes, WI: Lotus Press, 2007.

———. *Path of Fire and Light: Advanced Practices of Yoga*. 2 vols. Honesdale, PA: Himalayan Institute Press, 2007.

———. *Perennial Psychology of the Bhagavad-Gita*. Honesdale, PA: Himalayan Institute Press, 2007.

Rama, Swami, Rudolph Ballentine, and Swami Ajaya. *Yoga and Psychotherapy: The Evolution of Consciousness*. Honesdale, PA: Himalayan Institute Press, 1976.

Rettner, Rachel. "Epigenetics: Definitions and Examples." Live Science. June 24, 2013. www.livescience.com/37703-epigenetics.html

Roche, Lorin. *The Radiance Sutras: 112 Gateways to the Yoga of Wonder and Delight*. Boulder, CO: Sounds True, 2014.

Rosenberg, Stanley. *Accessing the Healing Power of the Vagus Nerve: Self-Help Exercises for Anxiety, Depression, Trauma, and Autism*. Berkeley, CA: North Atlantic Books, 2017.

Saraswati, Swami Satyasangananda. *Sri Vijanan Bhairava Tantra: The Ascent*. Yoga Publications Trust/Bihar School of Yoga, 2003.

Science of Consciousness. "Elmer E. Green Biography." http://www.consciousnessandbiofeedback.org/elmer-green-biography/.

Sih, G. C., and K. K. Tang. "On–Off Switching of Theta–Delta Brain Waves Related to Falling Asleep and Awakening." *Theoretical and Applied Fracture Mechanics* 63–64, February–April (2013): 1–17. doi.org/10.1016/j.tafmec.2013.03.001.

Somé, Sobonfu. *Women's Wisdom from the Heart of Africa*. Louisville, CO: Sounds True, 2007.

Stankovic, L. "Transforming Trauma: A Qualitative Feasibility Study of Integrative Restoration (iRest) Yoga Nidra on Combat-Related Post-traumatic Stress Disorder." *International Journal of Yoga Therapy* 21, no. 1 (2011): 23–37.

Stanley, Tracee. *Empowered Life: Soul Journal and Coloring Book*. Morrisville, NC: Lulu.com, 2017.

Stryker, Rod. *The Four Desires Workbook: Creating a Life of Purpose, Happiness, Prosperity, and Freedom*. New York: Delacorte Press, 2011.

Symphonic Mind. "What Are Brainwaves?" Brainworks. www.brainworks-neurotherapy.com/what-are-brainwaves. Accessed July 27, 2020.

Tantroktam Rātrisūktam: Praise of the Goddess Night Revealed in the Tantra. Nadiad, India: Dharmsinh Desai Institute of Technology, 2000.

Tejomayananda, Swami. *Divinising the Mind: Siva-sankalpa Suktam*. Mumbai, India: Chinmaya Prakashan, 2010.

Tigunait, Pandit Rajmani. *Living Tantra*. Lecture series. Yoga International, 2020. https://yogainternational.com/ecourse/living-tantra.

————. *The Practice of the Yoga Sutra: Sadhana Pada.* Honesdale, PA: Himalayan Institute, 2017.

————. *The Secret of the Yoga Sutra: Samadhi Pada.* Honesdale, PA: Himalayan Institute, 2014.

————, trans. *Shiva Sutra.* Honesdale, PA: Himalayan Institute Press, 2015.

Vieten, Cassandra, Helane Wahbeh, B. Rael Cahn, et al. "Future Directions in Meditation Research: Recommendations for Expanding the Field of Contemplative Science." PLoS ONE 13, no. 11 (2018): e0205740. doi.org/10.1371/journal.pone.0205740.

Walker, Matthew. *Why We Sleep: Unlocking the Power of Sleep and Dreams.* New York: Scribner, 2017.

Recommended Resources

THE GODDESS

Goddess Durgā and Sacred Female Power by Laura Amazzone
In Praise of the Goddess: The Devimahatmya and Its Meaning by Devadatta Kālī
Tantric Yoga and the Wisdom Goddesses by David Frawley
Tantroktam Rātrisūktam: Praise of the Goddess Night Revealed in the Tantra from the Devī Mahātmyam

YOGA SUTRAS

Living the Sutras: A Guide to Yoga Wisdom beyond the Mat by Amy Pearce-Hayden and Kelly DiNardo
The Practice of the Yoga Sutra: Sadhana Pada by Pandit Rajmani Tigunait
The Secret Power of the Yoga: A Woman's Guide to the Heart and Spirit of the Yoga Sutras by Nischala Joy Devi
Yoga Sutras of Patanjali: With the Exposition of Vyasa, Volume One, A Translation and Commentary by Pandit Arya
Yoga Sutras of Patanjali: With the Exposition of Vyasa, Volume Two by Swami Veda Bharati

HISTORY OF HARM IN YOGA NIDRA

Yoni Shakti (Revised Edition) by Uma Dinsmore-Tuli

YOGA NIDRA NEST CRAFTING

The Ritual of Rest course by Chanti Tacoronte-Perez;
www.yantrawisdom.com/rest

DEEP RELAXATION POSTURES

Restore and Rebalance: Yoga for Deep Relaxation by Judith Hanson Lasater

STATES OF CONSCIOUSNESS

OM the Eternal Witness: Secrets of the Mandukya Upanishad by Swami Rama

RELAXATION

*Accessing the Healing Power of the Vagus Nerve: Self-Help Exercises for Anxiety,
    Depression, Trauma, and Autism* by Stanley Rosenberg
The Relaxation Response by Dr. Herbert Benson

SUBTLE BODY ANATOMY

The Subtle Body: An Encyclopedia of Your Energetic Anatomy by Cyndi Dale
Yoga of the Subtle Body: A Guide to the Physical and Energetic Anatomy of Yoga
    by Tias Little

RACE-BASED TRAUMA

Decolonization Toolkit by Yoli Maya Yeh; www.yogawithyoli.com
*My Grandmother's Hands: Racialized Trauma and the Pathway to Mending
    Our Hearts and Bodies* by Resmaa Menakem
Radiant Rest podcast, episode 1 with Dr. Gail Parker
Restorative Yoga for Ethnic and Race-Based Stress and Trauma by Dr. Gail Parker

SANKALPA

Divinising the Mind by Swami Tejomayananda

The Four Desires: Creating a Life of Purpose, Happiness, Prosperity, and Freedom by Rod Stryker

RITUAL

Women's Wisdom from the Heart of Africa by Sobonfu Somé

SLEEP

Why We Sleep: Unlocking the Power of Sleep and Dreams by Matthew Walker

NEUROSCIENCE

The Brain That Changes Itself: Stories of Personal Triumph from the Frontiers of Brain Science by Norman Doidge

Breaking the Habit of Being Yourself: How to Lose Your Mind and Create a New One by Dr. Joe Dispenza

MANTRA

Mantra Yoga and Primal Sound: Secret of Seed (Bija) Mantras by David Frawley

Sacred Sound Lab with Sheela Bringi, https://www.sacredsoundlab.com

HEART-CENTERED PRACTICES

Vishoka Meditation: The Yoga of Inner Radiance by Pandit Rajmani Tigunait

About the Author

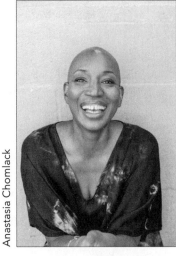

Anastasia Chomlack

Tracee Stanley was introduced to the practice of yoga nidra in 2001. She immediately recognized it as a healing salve for the world and began to incorporate it into her life as a way to balance the chaos of her career as a Hollywood film producer.

Tracee is a lineaged teacher with more than twenty years of study and practice in the Himalayan tradition, Tantra, and Sri Vidya. As a householder, she also understands the demands of life as an entrepreneur, wife, and stepmom, and it is with this lens that she shares her understanding of time-tested practices. Her effortless, accessible way of sharing ancient teachings has reached thousands as she travels across the world, teaching and sharing with the intention that everyone experiences their birthright of deep rest and awakening to their innate power and wisdom.